Biotechnology and the Food Supply

Proceedings of a Symposium

Food and Nutrition Board
Commission on Life Sciences
National Research Council

NATIONAL ACADEMY PRESS
Washington, D.C.   1988

NOTICE: The project that is the subject of this report was approved by the Governing Board of the National Research Council, whose members are drawn from the councils of the National Academy of Sciences, the National Academy of Engineering, and the Institute of Medicine.

This report has been reviewed by a group other than the authors according to procedures approved by a Report Review Committee consisting of members of the National Academy of Sciences, the National Academy of Engineering, and the Institute of Medicine.

The National Academy of Sciences is a private, nonprofit, self-perpetuating society of distinguished scholars engaged in scientific and engineering research, dedicated to the furtherance of science and technology and to their use for the general welfare. Upon the authority of the charter granted to it by the Congress in 1863, the Academy has a mandate that requires it to advise the federal government on scientific and technical matters. Dr. Frank Press is president of the National Academy of Sciences.

The National Academy of Engineering was established in 1964, under the charter of the National Academy of Sciences, as a parallel organization of outstanding engineers. It is autonomous in its administration and in the selection of its members, sharing with the National Academy of Sciences the responsibility for advising the federal government. The National Academy of Engineering also sponsors engineering programs aimed at meeting national needs, encourages education and research, and recognizes the superior achievements of engineers. Dr. Robert M. White is president of the National Academy of Engineering.

The Institute of Medicine was established in 1970 by the National Academy of Sciences to secure the services of eminent members of appropriate professions in the examination of policy matters pertaining to the health of the public. The Institute acts under the responsibility given to the National Academy of Sciences by its congressional charter to be an adviser to the federal government and, upon its own initiative, to identify issues of medical care, research, and education. Dr. Samuel O. Thier is president of the Institute of Medicine.

The National Research Council was organized by the National Academy of Sciences in 1916 to associate the broad community of science and technology with the Academy's purposes of furthering knowledge and advising the federal government. Functioning in accordance with general policies determined by the Academy, the Council has become the principal operating agency of both the National Academy of Sciences and the National Academy of Engineering in providing services to the government. The Council is administered jointly by both Academies and the Institute of Medicine. Dr. Frank Press and Dr. Robert M. White are chairman and vice chairman, respectively, of the National Research Council.

The work on which this publication is based was supported by the National Research Council Fund--a pool of private, discretionary, nonfederal funds that is used to support a program of Academy-initiated studies of national issues in which science and technology figure significantly. The Fund consists of contributions from a consortium of private foundations including the Carnegie Corporation of New York, the Charles E. Culpeper Foundation, the William and Flora Hewlett Foundation, the John D. and Catherine T. MacArthur Foundation, the Andrew W. Mellon Foundation, the Rockefeller Foundation, and the Alfred P. Sloan Foundation; the Academy Industry Program, which seeks annual contributions from companies that are concerned with the health of U.S. science and technology and with public policy issues with technological content; and the National Academy of Sciences and the National Academy of Engineering endowments.

The views expressed in this book are solely those of the individual authors and are not necessarily the views of the Food and Nutrition Board.

Copies available from:

Food and Nutrition Board
National Research Council
2101 Constitution Ave., NW
Washington, D.C. 20418

FOOD AND NUTRITION BOARD

KURT J. ISSELBACHER (Chairman), Harvard Medical School and Department of Gastroenterology, Massachusetts General Hospital, Boston, Massachusetts
RICHARD J. HAVEL (Vice Chairman), Cardiovascular Research Institute, University of California School of Medicine, San Francisco, California
HAMISH N. MUNRO (Vice Chairman), Human Nutrition Research Center on Aging, Tufts University, Boston, Massachusetts
WILLIAM E. CONNOR, Department of Medicine, Oregon Health Sciences University, Portland, Oregon
PETER GREENWALD, Division of Cancer Prevention and Control, National Cancer Institute, Bethesda, Maryland
M. R. C. GREENWOOD, Department of Biology, Vassar College, Poughkeepsie, New York
JOAN D. GUSSOW, Department of Nutrition Education, Teachers College, Columbia University, New York, New York
JAMES R. KIRK, Research and Development, Campbell Soup Company, Camden, New Jersey
BERNARD J. LISKA, Department of Food Science, Purdue University, West Lafayette, Indiana
REYNALDO MARTORELL, Food Research Institute, Stanford University, Stanford, California
WALTER MERTZ, Human Nutrition Research Center, Agricultural Research Service, U.S. Department of Agriculture, Beltsville, Maryland

MALDEN C. NESHEIM, Division of Nutritional Sciences, Cornell University, Ithaca, New York
RONALD C. SHANK, Department of Community and Environmental Medicine and Department of Pharmacology, University of California, Irvine, California
ROBERT H. WASSERMAN, Department/Section of Physiology, New York State College of Veterinary Medicine, Cornell University, Ithaca, New York
MYRON WINICK, Institute of Human Nutrition, College of Physicians and Surgeons, Columbia University, New York, New York
J. MICHAEL McGINNIS (Ex Officio), Office of Disease Prevention and Health Promotion, Department of Health and Human Services, Washington, D.C.
ARNO G. MOTULSKY (Ex Officio), Center for Inherited Diseases, University of Washington, Seattle, Washington

Staff

SUSHMA PALMER, Director, Food and Nutrition Board
FRANCES PETER, Editor, Commission on Life Sciences

PREFACE

Biotechnology and the food supply was the subject of the Food and Nutrition Board's annual symposium held on December 1, 1986, at the National Academy of Sciences in Washington, D.C. The papers presented at the symposium, and contained in this volume, address various aspects of this topic, including food production, food safety, and food quality.

Eleven years ago at the Asilomar conference on recombinant DNA, biotechnology and genetic engineering were in their infancy, and very few people really predicted or appreciated the overall impact that this new technology would have. For example, through biotechnology it has been possible to make plants resistant to drought, to develop vaccines against disabling viral diseases of animals, and as these proceedings indicate, to modify foods and the food supply both before and after harvest.

When we speak about biotechnology, we must include not only recombinant DNA techniques but also the techniques of producing monoclonal antibodies and the ability to grow cells in culture. When we refer to monoclonal antibodies, we are talking about very specific and selective proteins with great potential. They are so specific that they can be viewed as specific keys to a lock. Imagine all the doors with their locks and keys in the White House and in the Capitol. If the monoclonal antibodies were keys, they could be coded so specifically that one could have one antibody to fit only a single one of the many locks. Hence, they are very powerful tools that can be used to purify medically important materials such as hormones or vaccines. At the same time, they can be used to remove chemical or bacterial toxins to improve the quality of the food supply.

Tissue culture is also an important tool. For example, we can select individual cells such as plant cells, grow them into plants, or combine them with other types of plant cells to form hybrid or better quality plants or vegetables.

In essence, recombinant DNA techniques make possible the isolation of a specific gene of interest. For example, consider the gene for the production of growth hormone. After it is isolated, the gene can be attached to a transporter or a vehicle to permit that gene to enter a recipient cell such as a bacterium, plant cell, or animal cell. After its incorporation into the cell, the DNA is then able to make a cell with new properties. Thus, one can regard the recipient cell as source material, since, as it continues to function or multiply, it generates the production of pure growth hormone.

When we considered the tools of biotechnology at this symposium, we took into account not only the ways these tools are used today but also the ways they should be used in the future and the possible caveats in their use and application. In considering uses and misuses of recombinant DNA technology, some scientists have focused more on the negative rather than on the positive aspects; some I think have even reached the conclusion that recombinant DNA technology is really bad for society. This symposium was intended to present a balanced perspective on this overall important issue.

Kurt J. Isselbacher, M.D., <u>Chairman</u>
Food and Nutrition Board

CONTENTS

I BIOTECHNOLOGY: FOOD PRODUCTION AND NEW PRODUCT DEVELOPMENT

The Gene Revolution
  Albert Gore, Jr. 3
The Impact of Biotechnology on Food Production
  Ernest G. Jaworski 9
New Applications of Biotechnology in the Food Industry
  Robert H. Lawrence, Jr. 19

II BIOTECHNOLOGY: FOOD SAFETY AND NEW ROLES FOR TRADITIONAL INSTITUTIONS

Potential Food Safety Problems Related to New Uses of Biotechnology
  Jack Doyle 49
Biotechnology: Its Potential Impact on Interrelationships Among Agriculture, Industry, and Society
  Lawrence Busch and William B. Lacy 75

AUTHORS AND COAUTHORS 107

BIOTECHNOLOGY: FOOD PROTECTION AND NEW PRODUCT DEVELOPMENT

THE GENE REVOLUTION

Albert Gore, Jr.

I commend the Food and Nutrition Board for tackling this challenge. In America, we have long taken the food supply for granted. Now we appear to be taking biotechnology for granted as well--with little regard for the difficult questions it will raise. As a long-time advocate of new technologies, I would like to thank the FNB for making these issues a matter of public debate. The sooner we prepare ourselves for the potential social and economic impacts of biotechnology, the more promising its prospects will be.

As you know, the science of genetic engineering presents wondrous possibilities. It will enable us to develop hardier crop strains, bigger and better livestock breeds, and new miracle drugs. Genetically altered vaccines, growth hormones, and other new products could eventually make hunger obsolete--even as the world population continues to soar.

But many fear that the brave new world of biotechnology will also have a dark side. Some of the new crops and livestock we develop may have no natural enemies and will be genetically superior to their predecessors. New organisms could multiply wildly, like kudzu or the gypsy moth, crowding out everything else. In theory, a genetically altered crop strain could have some tragic flaw that might not become apparent until it was already in wide use.

No one knows for certain how great those risks are. The uncertainty and confusion that surround the environmental release of genetically altered organisms have allowed staunch opponents like Jeremy Rifkin to block the new technology at every turn. Unwilling to wait for the United States to sort out the regulatory muddle, some companies have tested organisms abroad. Angered by a rabies vaccine experiment near Buenos Aires, Argentina recently accused us of engaging in environmental imperialism. The Argentines believe that by conducting these tests on foreign soil, American companies run the risk of a biotechnological Bhopal.

Perhaps pressure from overseas will push us along. We can't afford to leave environmental release in limbo forever. Uncertainty hurts industry and regulators alike.

But the most lasting impact of biotechnology on the food supply may come not from something going wrong, but from everything going right. Sooner or later, every inventor--from Albert Einstein to Dr. Frankenstein--confronts the same questions: First, how do we make the thing work? Second, how do we keep it from working too well?

For every use of biotechnology there is a potential misuse. For every benefit, there is a potential hazard. The challenge is to know when we are about to go too far with the technology and when the drawbacks outweigh the advantages.

My biggest fear is not that by accident we will set loose some genetically defective Andromeda strain. Given our record in dealing with agriculture, we are far more likely to accidentally drown ourselves in a sea of excess grain. The Green Revolution made America the world's breadbasket, but it also brought on an age of intractable overproduction. Unless we plan more carefully, the Gene Revolution could do the same--on an even grander scale.

What is the price of progress? Will the supercow trample the small dairy farmer? Is the family farm about to be genetically altered out of existence? Meanwhile, will biotechnology help to feed the starving millions? Or will it leave the Third World behind to eat our dust?

Let's look first at the threat of overproduction. As you know, these are hard times down on the farm--and if anything, the prospects are worse. We live in an age of excess--excess capacity, that is. A worldwide glut, lackluster domestic markets, and misguided agricultural policies have put American farmers in a precarious financial position. Since 1982, the value of American farmland has plunged $150 billion. The farm bankruptcy rate has quadrupled. Farm debt now exceeds $200 billion-- more than the foreign debt of Brazil, Mexico, and Argentina combined.

From the standpoint of the small farmer, even the Green Revolution has been a mixed blessing. Increased agricultural efficiency forced many family farms out of business and left others hostage to the increasing volatility of glutted commodity markets.

How, then, can the small farmer possibly survive the Gene Revolution? The effect of genetic advances on production will dwarf the triumphs of the past two decades. Already, we have seen bovine growth hormone that can make cows produce up to 40% more milk. Scientists are working on supercows, superpigs, even supersized salmon. Other experiments have led to multiple births, more rapid growth, and higher resistance to disease. Unless we can somehow find a way to create very hungry superhumans, each of these advances may produce nothing but glut.

In the next few years, our capacity to expand the food supply will grow at an unprecedented rate. The Gene Revolution will do for animal products what the Green Revolution did for crop yields. Much to the chagrin of the farmers, it will have the same effect on food prices as well. Robert Kalter, an agricultural economist at Cornell, predicts that "the unparalleled speed and magnitude of the expected productivity gains" will flood commodity markets. As prices fall, he thinks the cost of maintaining price supports will rise so rapidly that the government may have to abandon the program.

Moreover, for the individual farmer, most of these new developments in biotechnology will be out of reach. The quarter million family-size farms in this country, which are already on the ropes, will be hard pressed to afford the high startup costs. After the ruinous expansion of farm debt in the 1970s, banks may be more reluctant to lend small farmers money for expensive new investments--and quicker to foreclose on them if anything goes wrong. Only the large farms will be able to afford a new technology, which if it works could drive their smaller competitors out of business. Biotechnology will be a hollow victory for science or for society if only the big guys survive to divide the spoils.

It doesn't have to be that way. With the right planning, biotechnology could be the salvation of the family farm rather than the death of it. One way or another, biotechnology will become a cornerstone of our future prosperity. The challenge is to make sure it will help those who need it--from the wheat grower in West Tennessee to the starving peasant farmer in Africa.

How can we turn this revolution into the common man's revenge? We can start by changing our approach to agricultural research. In our all-out rush to boost total production during the Green Revolution, we stopped worrying about producers. We almost forgot the small farmer, who needed cost-effective <u>applied</u> technology. The yield on a large farm in Iowa is 40 times that of a subsistence farm in Nigeria--not just because American farmers are more efficient but also because the world has yet to develop agricultural techniques that work on a small scale. Traditionally, 95% of all agricultural research has been geared toward agribusiness, to ever greater efficiencies of scale.

Today we're paying for that policy of bigger is better-- with bigger farm debts, a bigger price-support program, and big troubles for all but the biggest farms. We cannot afford to make that mistake again. Biotechnology can and ought to be a Great Equalizer, making a miraculous yield possible on even a small plot of land.

That should be an important goal of our research. Instead of rewarding agribusiness interests or distributing academic pork barrel, government grants should target the individual farmer. I hope we never see another U. S. Department of Agriculture study on how long Americans take to cook breakfast. We should worry instead about what

Americans are <u>eating</u> for breakfast and how the farmer can provide a cheap, tasty, and nutritious product.

Unless we consciously steer progress toward the little guy, it will trickle down too late to do much good. I would like to explore the possibility of a Biotechnology Extension Service that would offer technological assistance in agricultural areas. Biotechnology will bloom and grow only if it is affordable and easy to understand.

The government might also consider a Rural Development Bank to give small farmers low-interest loans for appropriate biotechnology. Eventually, we could apply our success in the Third World, so the areas that need progress most don't fall further behind.

Here at home, we can use our technological research to target the individual consumer. One biotech company (DNA Plant Technology) has begun to produce healthy snacks, such as carrots that are extra sweet and popcorn that tastes buttery without adding butter. Instead of continually trying to change people's diets, we may some day be able to take the dietary risk out of high-risk foods.

The Gene Revolution is still young and full of possibilities. It can bring on a brave new era--or just a lot more of the same old thing. The choice is ours. Will we sit back and watch the gap widen between rich and poor, North and South, the agribusinessman and family farmer? Or will we use this fabulous opportunity to leap ahead together?

In the years to come, government must learn to give people the tools to control their own destiny, make their own choices, and find their own way. Biotechnology is a key to that future. Let's make sure it ends up in the right hands.

THE IMPACT OF BIOTECHNOLOGY ON FOOD PRODUCTION

Ernest G. Jaworski

The application of recombinant DNA techniques to biological organisms, systems, and processes constitutes an exciting new biology that is being used to increase agricultural productivity and to improve the health of humans and animals. These advances coupled with those resulting from more traditional genetic and chemical approaches are having and will continue to have an enormous impact on the production of food throughout the world.

These applications could each be described in some depth, but this would require more pages than are available in this volume. Therefore, this paper focuses mainly on the most recent advances in the transformation of plants, even though the creation of transgenic animals is actively being explored at the fundamental and applied levels.

Advances in plant cell and tissue culture have made it possible in some cases to insert genetic information into the chromosome of an organism and then to regenerate whole plants from single cell cultures. Such techniques have been used to produce protoplasts, i.e., plant cells without a cell wall, which are useful in transformation. This significant development, coupled with the ability to clone pieces of functional DNA using bacterial systems and restriction endonuclease-generated DNA fragments, has provided the basic tools for the creation of transgenic plants. The key ingredient in the most recent advances in plant transformation resulted from the use of a naturally occurring bacterium (<u>Agrobacterium</u> <u>tumefaciens</u>) that has the capacity to insert its DNA stably into the chromosome of plant cells (Fraley et al., 1986). This system can be used in conjunction with plant cell culture to successfully produce whole plants containing foreign gene inserts.

CELL TRANSFORMATION SYSTEM

<u>Agrobacterium</u> <u>tumefaciens</u> contains a large Ti, or tumor-inducing, plasmid that in its wild form is capable of creating crown gall tumors in plants. The Ti plasmid can transfer a small portion of its DNA (T-DNA) and stably insert it into the nuclear DNA of the transformed cell. Since the T-DNA contains genetic information responsible for the synthesis of plant hormones as well as novel metabolites called opines, its transfer and insertion creates the crown gall tumor when these genes are expressed. Although the mechanisms by which these transfer and insertion processes take place are not well understood, it has been possible to take advantage of <u>Agrobacterium</u>'s properties to genetically engineer the Ti plasmid into a useful transforming vector. Intermediate vectors containing selectable antibiotic resistance markers for the introduction of foreign genes into the Ti plasmid have been constructed and the tumor-inducing properties of <u>Agrobacterium</u> deleted by removal of the plant hormone genes.

The neomycin phosphotransferase (NPT) coding sequences from a bacterial transposon (Tn5) were joined to the 5' and 3' regulatory sequences of nopaline synthase--a gene derived from the Ti plasmid, which is known to be constitutively expressed in plants (Fraley et al., 1986). This chimeric gene confers resistance to kanamycin, an aminoglycoside antibiotic that is lethal to plant cells. Thus this chimeric gene construct provided a selectable marker for the transformation vector.

Direct cloning approaches using the Ti plasmids were not practical. It was therefore necessary to create intermediate or shuttle vectors either to integrate with a resident Ti plasmid by recombination or to replicate independently of the Ti plasmid as transvectors. The integrated vector was then used for the transfer of a number of foreign genes into Agrobacterium cells. The characteristics of these plasmids include a segment of the pBR322 DNA for replication in Escherichia coli, a portion of a Ti plasmid (pTiT37) containing the functional nopaline synthase gene for ease in scoring transformed plant cells, a streptomycin/spectinomycin resistance determinant from Tn7 for selection in Agrobacterium, a portion of DNA from another Ti plasmid (pTiA6) to provide homology for recombination with a resident octopine-type plasmid in A. tumefaciens, a synthetic multilinker containing unique sites for gene insertion, and the chimeric kanamycin resistance gene (NOS/NPT II/NOS). These plasmids and derivatives were introduced into A. tumefaciens by conjugation procedures and homologous recombination between the plasmid and the wild-type octopine Ti plasmid to produce cointegrates (Fraley et al., 1986). Although this system was useful for the study of gene expression and inheritance of traits, it was not sufficiently efficient for routine production of transformed plants. A subsequent series of derivatives led to the formation of a variant and selectable T-DNA system, which was highly efficient in its transformation frequency (Fraley et al., 1986).

PLANT TRANSFORMATION SYSTEM

Initially, an in vitro transformation was developed by incubating plant protoplasts directly in A. tumefaciens cell suspension (Fraley et al., 1986). Protoplasts were prepared from a variety of leaf tissues by conventional enzyme digestion. The bacteria attached to the protoplasts during cell wall regeneration and subsequently transferred the T-DNA into the plant cells by an unknown mechanism. Such cells were easily identified within 3 weeks by selection for kanamycin resistance.

Since the protoplast system had a number of technical drawbacks, an improved alternative procedure was developed to obviate problems in the isolation and regeneration of protoplasts. The modification involved cutting disks from leaves and infecting them with Agrobacterium. These disks were then placed on nutrient agar. Subsequently, callus formation was observed around the circumference of the disks. Within 3 to 4 weeks, plant regeneration occurred under appropriate conditions.

Stable maintenance and expression of foreign genes (kanamycin resistance) were demonstrated in cells and plants derived from either the protoplast cocultivation or leaf disk systems. Subsequent progeny seed derived from the transformed plants inherited the kanamycin resistance in a simple Mendelian manner.

GENE EXPRESSION

The development of a transformation system for the stable and heritable introduction and expression of a foreign gene provided a tool for the analysis of gene expression in general. The first study in this effort involved light-regulated, tissue-specific gene coding for the small subunit of ribulose-1,5-bisphosphatecarboxylase (RuBPss) from peas (Fraley et al., 1986). The investigators demonstrated that the genomic clone for pea RuBPss could be introduced into petunia cells by cocultivation with A. tumefaciens. Molecular analyses of transformed cells revealed that the small subunit gene of the pea was indeed expressed in the petunia under the control of its own promoter and was regulated by light in a manner identical to that seen for the endogenous gene in peas. The pea RuBPss retained its tissue-specific pattern of expression in leaves derived from regenerated transformed petunia plants. Subsequent studies using in vivo radiolabeling, followed by immunoprecipitation of ribulose-1, 5-bisphosphatecarboxylase, demonstrated that the heterologous RuBPss protein of the peas could be separated from the endogenous petunia RuBPss, thereby indicating that the pea RuBPss protein was correctly processed in vivo by petunia chloroplast (Fraley et al., 1986). In vivo pea RuBPss was also recovered from the holoenzyme, which was immunoselected with the petunia antilarge subunit antibody, indicating that the small subunit of the pea could form a hybrid holoenzyme assembly with large subunits of the petunia.

Two mammalian genes were also demonstrated to be expressed in plant cells. A cDNA clone encoding α-human chorionogonadotropin (α-hCG) under the control of the cauliflower mosaic virus 35s promoter and a mouse cDNA clone encoding a methotrexate-insensitive dihydrofolate reductase (DHFR) gene also under the control of the cauliflower mosaic 35s promoter expressed their gene products in transformed petunia cells. The results with α-hCG and the mouse DHFR indicate the broad utility of the Agrobacterium system for the study of gene expression and regulation.

Finally, the transfer of a legume storage protein gene into the petunia resulted in the tissue-specific accumulation of the storage protein in the seeds of the transformed plants. A cDNA clone encoding the soybean 7s α'-conglycinin protein was engineered into an appropriate Agrobacterium plasmid and transferred into petunia cells (Fraley et al., 1986). Analysis of subsequent petunia seeds indicated that there was regulated expression of the soybean storage protein gene in the petunia seed. This exciting model system for storage protein expression should permit the determination of the structural sequences required for protein translocation, glycosylation, and processing as well as the study of the regulatory sequences essential for seed-specific expression.

TECHNOLOGY APPLICATIONS

Plants

In the past 3 years, the gene transfer systems described above have led to important new insights into gene regulation and protein transport in plants. The basic applications of this technology should provide a means for developing deeper understandings of the specific promoter/enhancer DNA sequences involved in gene expression and fundamental information on cis and trans gene regulation.

Of specific interest, however, has been the recent demonstration of agronomically significant transformations involving the generation of herbicide-tolerant, insect-resistant, and viral disease-resistant plants. The herbicide N-(phosphonomethyl)glycine, or glyphosate, is the active ingredient in Roundup®. It inhibits the aromatic biosynthetic pathway at its sixth step; namely, enolpyruvylshikimate-3-phosphate (EPSP) synthase (Fraley et al., 1986). This pathway is involved in the biosynthesis of phenylalanine, tyrosine, and tryptophan, and when the pathway is inhibited at the EPSP synthase level, the formation of these essential amino acids ceases. Early studies indicated that overproduction of a bacterial EPSP synthase in bacteria results in herbicide tolerance (Fraley et al., 1986). Subsequent efforts led to the development of a chimeric gene construct consisting of a petunia EPSP synthase cDNA flanked by the cauliflower mosaic 35s 5' promoter and the nopaline synthase, 3' regulatory regions. Transformation of petunia cells with this construct resulted in herbicide resistance and the overproduction of EPSP synthase 30- to 60-fold. Plants regenerated from these cell lines were found to be tolerant to Roundup® when sprayed at concentrations of 0.9 kg/hectare. Control plants were killed when sprayed with the herbicide at 0.22 kg/hectare. Similar strategies are currently being used to create plants tolerant to a number of other herbicides such as atrazine, the imidazolidinone series, sulfonylureas, and phosphonotricine.

Within the past few years, numerous crop plants, including canola, tomato, potato, tobacco, lettuce, sugar beets, and poplar, have become amenable to the transformation technologies involving <u>Agrobacterium</u>. On the basis of these rapid advances, it can be expected that practical demonstrations of the system are forthcoming. Within the past year, field tests were initiated with genetically engineered tobacco that is resistant to atrazine.

The creation of a transformation vector for the production of viral disease resistance in plants was recently reported by the R. Beachy Group at Washington University (Powell-Abel et al., 1986). The transformation system described above was used to insert and express the tobacco mosaic virus (TMV) coat protein gene in both tobacco and tomato plants. The coat protein gene was engineered into a plasmid similar to the one described for herbicide tolerance. Both tobacco and tomato plants transformed with the coat protein gene were found either to be resistant to TMV infection or to demonstrate significant delays (weeks) in symptomology following infection. Control plants always demonstrated severe symptoms within days following inoculation with the virus. This is one of the first demonstrations of the genetic engineering of disease resistance in plants. Studies by AgroCetus have recently been carried into the field assessment stage with tobacco genetically engineered to be tolerant of soil-borne <u>Agrobacterium</u> infections.

Finally, a Belgian company, Plant Genetic Sciences, has recently demonstrated that the <u>Bacillus thuringiensis</u> (B.t.) toxin gene could be inserted into the Ti plasmid system and expressed in tobacco at sufficient concentrations to protect the tobacco plants from attack by the tobacco hornworm. This was the first demonstration of engineering to protect a plant against insect damage by using biotechnology.

These results demonstrate that single gene traits can be successfully introduced into plants for expression and that they can function at potentially economic levels. On the basis of these findings, it can be anticipated that useful single gene traits will also be inserted into plants in combination with other functionally important single gene traits. Furthermore, the stage has now been set for the examination of other genetic traits.

MICROORGANISMS

Transformations of microorganisms that colonize plants are also expected to be useful in enhancing the productivity of plants. For example, transformed <u>Pseudomonas florescens</u>, which is a natural colonizer of roots in such major crops as corn and soybeans, has been engineered to carry and express the <u>Bacillus thuringiensis</u> toxin gene mentioned earlier. Greenhouse tests have indicated that such microorganisms are capable of protecting the root systems of corn plants from attack by certain soil-borne insects. Similar advances can be expected in the development of both root-colonizing and leaf-colonizing organisms, which will protect plants from diseases, pests, and environmental stresses. Laboratory and greenhouse studies certainly promise that such organisms will effectively aid in plant productivity. Much further work will be needed to develop performance characteristics for these microorganisms under normal field conditions and soil types, and a special need exists to generate more basic data on the ecology of these microbes. In this regard, the E. coli lacZY genes (coding for β-galactosidase and lactose permease) have been engineered into Pseudomonas florescens to create a well-marked microorganism for microbial ecology research. The microorganism contains four marker characteristics that make it possible to isolate it from soil samples and detect it at levels of one bacterium per gram of soil. The characteristics of the engineered pseudomonad include its fluorescent properties, natural rifampicin resistance, ability to grow on a simple lactose media, and detection by the X-gal chromogenic dye. Thus this microorganism provides a very sensitive, selectable tracking system that should be extremely useful in ecological studies under natural environmental conditions.

FUTURE NEEDS AND EXPECTATIONS

The applications of genetic engineering and modern molecular biology have provided us with the ability to insert novel genetic traits into plants and into microorganisms that interact with plants. It can be predicted that this technology will have an impact on the production of food and on the efficiency of crop production throughout the world, since weeds, insects, and diseases create enormous losses in food production. Advances in the more qualitative traits in our food supply can also be anticipated and are in fact receiving attention at present. For example, extensive efforts are being devoted to the development of higher levels of solids in tomatoes by enhancing the concentration of natural polymers normally present in tomatoes. Protein engineering may well see its first application in simple amino acid codon shifts in seed storage proteins to enhance their content of lysine (e.g., in corn) or methionine (e.g., in soybeans). Gene engineering techniques may also be useful in improving the yield of protein levels in a variety of crops, especially forage crops. Site-directed mutagenesis may be applied to the creation of more stable proteins for storage purposes. The loss of food products and gains in storage may be reduced by subsequent genetic engineering of the crops to create disease- and insect-resistant products. We now have the technologies and tools to approach some of these important food supply issues, but we should consider some of the future needs that could help advance progress more rapidly.

Technical hurdles that still remain include cell culture procedures to broaden the base of crop species that can be regenerated, especially from protoplasts. Interestingly, a recent announcement by Japanese and French scientists indicates that it is now possible to regenerate rice plants from protoplast cultures. New transformation systems are needed, especially for monocot transformation. Other methods for the transfer of DNA into plant cells are being investigated, and there are indications that methods such as electroporation, microinjection, laser treatment, and the use of gemini virus vectors will soon have an impact on this field. Gene structure and function will continue to receive attention, especially with reference to the regulatory sequences affecting gene expression at the developmental and tissue-specific level. Among the most practical needs for the modification of our food supply will be the identification of additional agronomically important genes that can be used to create stress- and pest-tolerant plants.

At present, the lack of knowledge about the basic biochemistry of plant systems remains one of the major limiting factors in the advancement and exploitation of the technology described. This knowledge is vital for our understanding of the genetic components involved in achieving such traits as frost tolerance, heat tolerance, drought tolerance, metal tolerance, disease resistance, and insect tolerance. Incentives have been provided to improve this situation, but additional resources must be directed toward improving plant tissue culture and regeneration; novel transformation systems; understanding of gene structure organization and function; the selection, isolation, and characterization of agronomically important genes; and the development of unique plant-breeding techniques. Only then will the sociological and economic impacts of these exciting technologies and tools be fully realized.

REFERENCES

Fraley, R.T., S.G. Rogers, and R.B. Horsch. 1986. Genetic transformation in higher plants. CRC Crit. Rev. Plant Sci. 4(1):1-46.

Powell-Abel, P., R.S. Nelson, B. De, N. Hoffman, S.G. Rogers, R.T. Fraley, and R.N. Beachy. 1986. Delay of disease development in transgenic plants that express the tobacco mosaic virus coat protein gene. Science 232:738-743.

NEW APPLICATIONS OF BIOTECHNOLOGY IN THE FOOD INDUSTRY

Robert H. Lawrence

In the past several years, biotechnology in the food industry has been the central theme of numerous scientific reviews, national and international symposia, and several major reference works (Earle, 1984; Harlander and Labuza, 1986; Jarvis and Holmes, 1982; Kirsop, 1985; Knorr, 1987; Knorr and Sinskey, 1985; Moo-Young et al., 1985; Rehm and Reed, 1983). Reports of significant advances have come from the full spectrum of biotechnology research and development resources: universities and institutes as well as genetic "biotiques" and large food corporations. Important business alliances continue to be formed on a worldwide scale, linking advanced biotechnology research skills with large producers and marketers of food products, principally in the United States, Japan, the United Kingdom, and Europe. These alliances include Amgen/Kodak, CalBio/American Home Products, Genentech/Lilly, Genentech/Corning (Genencor), Interferon/Anheuser-Busch, Molecular Genetics/Upjohn, Synergen/Procter & Gamble, American Cyanamid/Pioneer Hi-Bred, Dupont/Advanced Genetic Sciences, W. R. Grace/Cetus (Agricetus), Hoechst/Harvard, Monsanto/Genentech, Monsanto/Washington University/Rockefeller University, Roche/Agrigenetics, Beatrice/Ingene, Campbell/DNA Plant Technology (DNAP), Campbell/Calgene, CPC/Enzyme Biosystems, Kraft/DNAP, General Foods/DNAP, Kellogg/Agrigenetics, Heinz/ARCO, McCormick/Native Plants, Inc., Molson/Allelix, RJR-Nabisco/Escagen, and Seagram/

Biotechnica. Corporate boards and strategic planning groups of major food companies now understand the language of biotechnology and can perceive its utility and value; this has been the case with their corporate research departments for years. One thing is clear: The excitement and enthusiasm for biotechnology so characteristic of the pharmaceutical and medical areas in the early 1980s have now begun to hit the food industry with increasing force, and this momentum will likely establish this industry as the largest commercial arena for biotechnology. Companies involved include Archer Daniels Midland, American Home Products, Beatrice, Campbell, Cargill, Corn Products Company, Coors, Chr. Hansen's Laboratory, Firmenich, General Foods, Heinz, Hunt-Wesson, Kraft, LaBatt, McCormick, Nestle, Pillsbury, Purdue, Procter & Gamble, Ralston, RJR-Nabisco, Staley, Unilever, and Universal Foods.

At least three important factors are responsible for this. First, in pharmaceuticals, the feasibility of the biotechnology promise has been established and the commercial reduction to practice (i.e., commercial application) is in place--in the marketplace! This was achieved by using many of the same technical concepts and strategies currently envisioned for food industry applications. Second, key advancements in technology continue to be made, principally in molecular genetics, cell technologies, computer-aided protein engineering, bioreactor design, and biosensor/diagnostic technology. These advancements have substantially redefined the technical skills base and broadened the potential applications of biotechnology to foods. Third, within the food industry, reports of successful new applications of biotechnology (e.g., those reported here) add confidence to the prediction that biotechnology may well be the next key source of competitive leverage at the corporate and international levels, and may be the most important single technical consideration in consolidation strategies.

The following paragraphs are a review of new applications of biotechnology in each of the following food-related areas: enzymes, including the processing of cheese; fermentation, including brewing and wine making; agricultural raw materials (e.g., crop plants, meat, poultry, fish) with improved functionality; and plant cell bioreactors for food ingredient production.

ENZYMES

Food Industry Uses

A recent report on the U.S. market for enzymes indicated total sales of $185 million in 1985, 58% of which was in the food industry (Charles Kline & Co., 1986). Of the classes of enzymes used by the food industry, the proteases and carbohydrases account for most of this market. The predominant protease sold is rennin (chymosin), which is used in cheese-making processes to coagulate milk to form curds. Of the carbohydrases, those used in cornstarch processing (the so-called starch enzymes α-amylase, glucoamylase, and glucose isomerase) account for 85% of sales. The other enzymes have diverse applications, including flavor development (e.g., lipases in cheese making) (Arbige et al., 1986), improvement of extractions (e.g., pectinases in juice processing) (Kilara, 1982), and modification of food functionality (e.g., α-amylases in retarding bread staling) (Boyce, 1986).

The technology for improvement of food enzyme production by genetic engineering is clearly in place (Lin, 1986). Genes for many of the important food industry enzymes have been cloned (Meade et al., 1987), and gene transfer systems that permit introduction and expression in generally recognized as safe (GRAS) organisms have been developed (Lin, 1986). Two recent, important applications of genetic engineering to enzyme production are α-amylase and chymosin.

α-Amylase: High Fructose Corn Syrup Industry.

The first petition to the Food and Drug Administration (FDA) to affirm the GRAS status of a food-processing enzyme produced by recombinant DNA techniques was for α-amylase. This landmark petition was filed by CPC International, Inc., on July 9, 1984.

α-Amylase is the enzyme used in the first step in the production of high-fructose corn syrup (HFCS), a widely used nutritive sweetener derived from cornstarch. The HFCS process was first developed in the United States between 1968 and 1972 by the Clinton Corn Processing Co. (Lloyd and Horwath, 1985) and involves three sequential

enzymatic steps. First, raw cornstarch is liquefied by
α-amylase hydrolysis to yield partially degraded starch
chains called dextrins. The dextrins are then hydrolyzed
by glucoamylase, which cleaves both the α-1,6 and α-1,4
glucosidic linkages to give corn syrup (glucose). This
glucose hydrolysate is refined and then isomerized by
immobilized glucose isomerase to give a mixture of glucose
and fructose (42%) known as HFCS. This last step was
commercialized in 1972 and represents the first
large-scale use of an immobilized enzyme permitting a
continuous process with significant cost reduction (Casey,
1977). The 42% HFCS can then be further purified
to yield second-generation syrups of 55% and 90% fructose
(Coker and Venkatasubramanian, 1985).

The market for HFCS has grown dramatically. U.S.
consumption increased from 2.3 kg/per person in 1975 to
20 kg/per person in 1985 (Newsome, 1986). Today, production exceeds 4.54 billion kg annually. HFCS is used in
many processed food products and is the principal
nutritive sweetener of the soft drink industry. Grant
(1986) recently discussed CPC's genetically engineered
α-amylase and its GRAS affirmation petition with the
FDA. His objective was to use Bacillus subtilis as a host
system for the commercial production of a thermostable
form of α-amylase that CPC had developed from Bacillus
stearothermophilus (Ishii et al., 1981)--an organism given
GRAS status by FDA (Figure 1). This heat- and acid-stable
form of α-amylase is important for low-cost production of
HFCS. Its production in B. subtilis was desired because
of the ease with which B. subtilis can be used in
commercial fermentations.

According to CPC's petition, the strain designated as
B. subtilis ATCC 39,705 was genetically derived from an
asporogenic variety of B. subtilis ATCC 39,701, which
lacked α-amylase, by introducing genetic material from
B. stearothermophilus ATCC 39,709 for α-amylase production. The genetically engineered B. subtilis contains
DNA from a plasmid vector designated as pCPC720. The
plasmid consists of a 2.4-kb portion of DNA comprising the
α-amylase gene from B. stearothermophilus and a portion
of DNA from plasmid pUB110 required for replication of the new plasmid. pCPC720 does not contain the
kanamycin resistance marker of pUB110, and transformed
host cells are not resistant to kanamycin.

- A Petition for the Affirmation of the GRAS Status of Alpha-Amylase Derived from *Bacillus subtilis* ATCC 39,705
  - Filed July 1984 by CPC International
  - Proposed commercial product: alpha-amylase G995 as a cell-free broth containing a thermostable form of enzyme

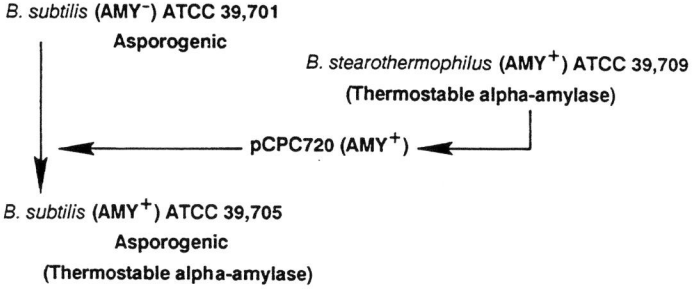

FIGURE 1 Genetically engineered α-amylase.

The CPC petition presents data characterizing the enzyme and recombinant organism to show that the genetically engineered enzyme is equivalent in every respect to that produced by B. stearothermophilus and to establish the safety of the recombinant product. The enzymes would be used in the HFCS process only and would not be present in the food product.

Regarding the CPC petition, Grant urged, "We need to have scientifically based regulatory decisions, and we need to have responsible industry actions. . . . Because this is the first of potentially many such petitions being reviewed by FDA with respect to a recombinant microorganism, the FDA has to be very careful and precise. The FDA ruling on our petition will set the policy for future rulings" (Grant, 1986, p. 22). That is no doubt the case: CPC in September was awarded a patent covering the genetic engineering of B. subtilis to produce a thermostable pullulanase (Coleman and McAlister, 1986). There are many similar developments, as shown in the following two examples.

Chymosin (Rennin): Dairy Industry. Another enzyme that has been the focus of considerable genetic engineering research is chymosin, the active component of rennet used in the dairy industry to coagulate milk to form curds in the cheese-making process. Chymosin is an endoprotease that is highly specific in the hydrolysis of peptide in bonds in the V-fold of kappa-casein of milk, resulting in the destabilization of casein micelles and subsequent curd formation. Commercial sources are calf rennet extracted from the fourth stomach of young suckling calves and microbial rennets principally from the fungi <u>Mucor miehei</u>, <u>M. pusillus</u>, or <u>Endothia parasitica</u>. These fungi produce chymosin with slight differences in milk-clotting properties, and in heat and pH stability, as well as a different coagulation/proteolysis ratio from that of chymosin from calf sources. Thus, a demand exists for chymosin similar to calf rennet for use in the production of quality cheeses. The opportunity for microbial production of calf rennet chymosin has led several companies to develop strategies to clone the gene for chymosin from cDNA libraries derived from calf stomach mRNA and to achieve expression of the heterologous gene in various host organisms (Figure 2). In vivo, chymosin is

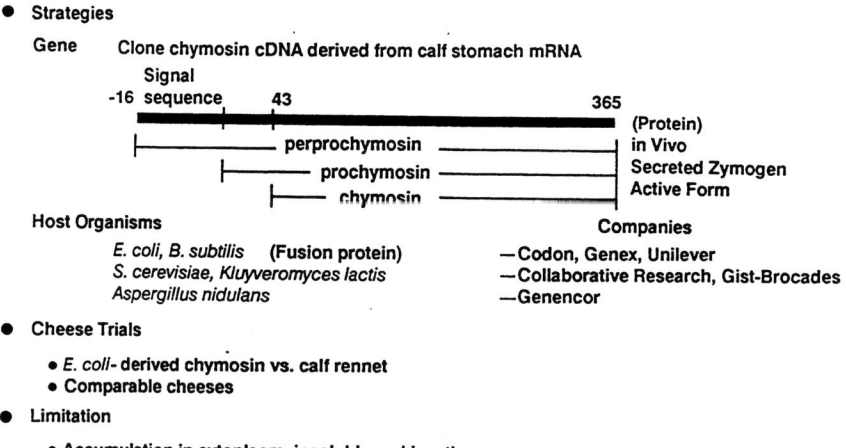

FIGURE 2 Genetically engineered chymosin production.

produced as preprochymosin, which is secreted as the zymogen, prochymosin. In low-pH solutions, prochymosin is autocatalytically cleaved to chymosin (McGuire, 1986).

Escherichia coli-produced chymosin has several limitations (Pitcher, 1986). The enzyme accumulates in the cytoplasm, requiring an expensive and low-yield process to derive the active enzyme. Two alternative host systems have been used: the so-called supersecretor strains of yeast (used by Collaborative Research, Inc.) and the filamentous fungi (used by Genencor, Inc.). The Genencor strategy for Aspergillus production of bovine chymosin (Heyneker et al., 1986; W.H. Pitcher, Genencor, personal communication, 1986) involved the use of heterologous gene constructions in A. nidulans transformants, which secrete the gene product.

Plasmid constructions consisted of the control regions of the A. niger glucoamylase gene coupled to either bovine prochymosin or preprochymosin cDNA with a glucoamylase terminator. A. nidulans transformants secreted chymosin, which was similar to authentic bovine chymosin in molecular weight and specific activity. Cheese trials using these chymosin preparations are being evaluated (Pitcher, 1986). Thus, commercial production of chymosin similar to calf rennet appears to be technically feasible.

Other applications of genetic engineering to enzyme production for the food industry include: lactase, to break down milk lactose; lipase and esterase, to develop cheese flavor; pectinase, to improve yield, reduce viscosity, and enhance clarification in fruit juice processing and wine making; protease, to serve as a malt substitute when used with barley; and carbohydrases, to facilitate carbohydrate metabolism in low-calorie beer production.

FERMENTATION

Brewing

Yocum (1986) of BioTechnica International has reported the development of a genetic engineering procedure suitable for polyploid industrial yeast (Saccharomyces cerevisiae) strains used in brewing. A new set of plasmids for industrial yeast transformation was developed;

these plasmids integrated the G418 resistance marker and targeted it for insertion at the HO (homothallism) locus. Multiple insertions were accomplished by a process that leaves the gene of interest integrated into the HO target locus but jettisons the G418 resistance gene. Yeasts transformed in this manner contain the new genes stably integrated into their chromosomes at homologous loci but with no remaining E. coli DNA sequences. For details of the plasmid contractions, refer to Figures 1 and 2 of Yocum (1986).

The BioTechnica group has demonstrated the commercial feasibility of this genetic engineering procedure in Saccharomyces for the production of light beer. BioTechnica cloned the gene coding for glucoamylase from A. niger and inserted the gene into brewing yeast. The glucoamylase expressed by the yeast during fermentation breaks down the soluble starch to glucose; this is metabolized by the yeast, resulting in a lower calorie beer without requiring the use of added enzyme preparations.

Wine Making

Snow (1985) has recently proposed a strategy for genetic engineering of industrial yeast strains used in wine making to introduce the capability for malolactic fermentation. The primary fermentation that occurs in wine making is achieved through the use of yeast to convert sugar to alcohol. A secondary fermentation may be allowed to occur, particularly during production of red wines, which is catalyzed by bacteria in the genera Leuconostoc, Lactobacillus, and Pediococcus. During this secondary fermentation, malic acid is converted to lactic acid, which causes a decrease in wine acidity, brings finished wine into better acid balance, and develops more desirable flavor complexity. Procedures used to encourage the malolactic fermentation may increase the risk of wine quality loss. They also increase the costs of wine production.

In the strategy proposed by Snow (1985) and experimentally investigated (Williams et al., 1984), the malolactic gene of Lactobacillus delbrueckii was introduced into a laboratory yeast strain. When this yeast was used to make wine in a trial fermentation, the malolactic gene was expressed and limited malate conversion occurred. Thus, the feasibility of this approach appears to have been demonstrated. Obviously, the yeast gene transfer system developed by BioTechnica would be of value in this approach.

AGRICULTURAL RAW MATERIALS

New applications of biotechnology are leading to notable improvements in yield and productivity in crop plants and animals (Jaworski, see paper in this volume). Crops may be specifically improved for functional attributes, such as nutrition, flavor, texture, and processibility. These improvements result in added value to the food processor as well as to the consumer.

Crop Plants

Figure 3 gives a food industry perspective of plant biotechnology. This discussion focuses on three areas: the central role of modern breeding strategies in crop development, new genetic tools and how they influence breeding strategies, and the functional attributes of crops along with the concept of utilization-side genetics and added value.

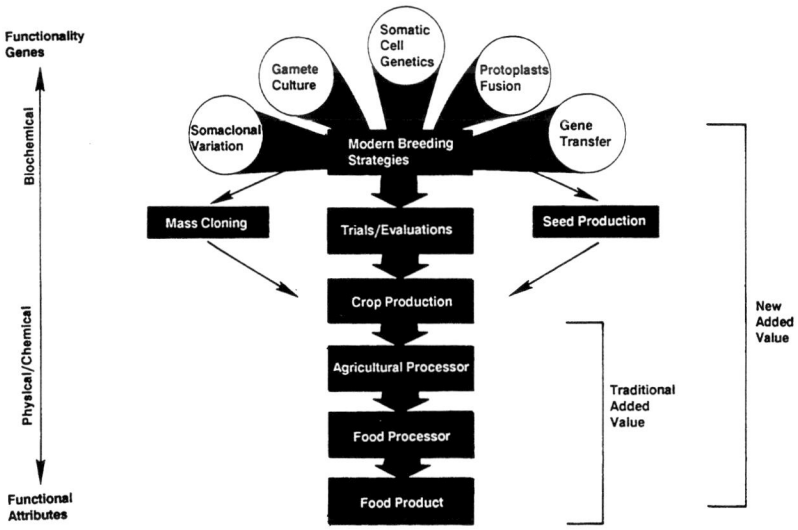

FIGURE 3 Plant biotechnology--food industry perspective.

Genetic Improvement Strategies. Most contemporary approaches to crop improvement are centered on modern breeding strategies that use a wide range of genetic tools and germplasm resources to generate genetic variability and diversity for traits of interest and to construct genotypes with new gene combinations from which new plant varieties are developed and then selected through a series of trials and evaluations. To be effective in their critical strategic role, contemporary plant breeders must be proficient in the application of an array of genetic techniques, including several new technologies that are only now being integrated into plant breeding programs. These technologies have brought about a dramatic reorientation of the plant breeders' approach to the introduction of new genes into existing varieties and have greatly expanded the potential sources from which new, useful genes can be accessed. Conventional germplasm resources, including valuable wild plant populations, will remain a primary gene source. Techniques that facilitate intergeneric gene transfer will increase the importance of these germplasm resources. However, accessibility to genes from outside the plant kingdom (e.g., from bacteria and animals) is now possible and will require that plant breeders adopt a broader, interdisciplinary perspective.

New hybridization systems for production of hybrid seeds are being developed; these involve cellular level manipulation of organellar genomes for cytoplasmic male sterility (Cocking, 1985) and the introduction of genes controlling self-incompatibility (Nasrallah and Nasrallah, 1985). New hybrid seed production schemes have also been developed; these involve cloned parent lines produced by tissue culture techniques (Lawrence and Hill, 1982, 1983). The ability to clone plants in large scale through somatic embryogenesis (Lawrence, 1981) and encapsulation to form synthetic seeds (Lutz et al., 1985; Redenbaugh et al., 1986) allow crops to be produced from unique genotypes, which cannot be economically reproduced through seeds. Thus, new options for crop establishment must be considered in developing breeding strategies.

Plant breeding programs make extensive use of trials and evaluations, typically in greenhouses and field plots, for the characterization of genotypes and for making selections that will be subject to breeding advancement or released for agricultural use. Under development are several diagnostic tools that permit evaluations and selections to be made in the laboratory (Frey, 1984). These tools include isozyme analysis and protein electrophoresis; DNA probes, molecular markers, and restriction fragment-length polymorphisms (RFLPs); and immunodiagnostics. Applications of these techniques in plant breeding are of value in the attainment of several objectives: (1) breeding for quantitative traits; (2) varietal identification and purity checks of seed lots; (3) screening for qualitative traits through marker linkage; (4) variety and genotype characterization for patent and Plant Variety Protection Certificate applications; (5) predictions of combining ability to improve breeding productivity; and (6) characterization of the expression of genes introduced by molecular techniques (Frey, 1984).

New Genetic Techniques. Several of the new genetic techniques currently being applied to plant breeding significantly extend the potential to manipulate crops genetically with greater efficiency and precision. These technologies include somaclonal variation, somatic cell genetics, gamete culture, protoplast fusion, and molecular approaches to gene transfer (Figure 3).

Although a considerable research effort in fundamental cellular and molecular biology has been required to develop these techniques as practical genetic tools, their strategic value in breeding must be considered within the context of the specific breeding objectives for a particular crop. A successful crop improvement program will generally require a balance in the use of more conventional approaches with predictable outcome, combined with more advanced tools with higher risks and less predictable utility. Both require a clear definition of traits targeted for improvement and a careful assessment of their commercial value.

All the following techniques rely heavily on the universal capability of plant cells and tissues to be grown and manipulated in vitro. Literature on this subject constitutes an extensive knowledge base. The value of plant cell and tissue culture lies in the ability not just to access molecular and cellular genetic strategies, but also to use them in a practical way. The key is the capability to regenerate intact plants containing new genetic capabilities that can be linked back into conventional plant breeding--the mechanism for achieving commercial value.

Somaclonal variation is a commonly observed phenomenon in plants regenerated from cells or tissues cultured in vitro. The genetic variability obtained is believed to be a combination of genetic changes that occurred in the original plant tissues or mutations induced in the tissue culture cycle. Evans and Sharp (1986) have reviewed the unique aspects of the somaclonal variation process and its practical utility in plant breeding. These aspects include the following: (1) The frequency of genetic variation is significantly higher than spontaneous mutation. (2) Genetic mosaics occur at a low frequency. (3) A somaclonal variant can generally be genetically stabilized in one generation. (4) Deleterious genetic changes are usually eliminated by the stringency of the regeneration event. (5) Cytoplasmic genetic changes have been observed. (6) Dominant as well as recessive mutant alleles are generated. Somaclonal variation thus appears to be an efficient method to generate useful genetic variability in several crop plants, notably tomatoes (Evans and Sharp, 1983) and wheat (Larkin et al., 1984).

Recently, Scowcroft and colleagues (1985) reported on the genetic and molecular analysis of somaclonal variants in wheat. They observed many genetic changes: increase in ploidy, gross chromosomal rearrangements, translocations, and single nucleotide substitutions. New variants not obtainable by other approaches were observed for several genetic loci. In addition, a high frequency of translocation among chromosomes was shown to be a useful mechanism to introgress alien genes into commercial varieties. Obviously, under certain conditions, the cell culture cycle can be like a genomic earthquake and may generate a wide array of variations.

Somatic cell genetic methods also rely on cell culture-generated variability. An additional step is included to permit selection for specific traits at the cellular level. This approach has been useful in the generation of traits for tolerance to toxic selection agents, such as herbicides (Miller and Hughes, 1980;

Shaner and Anderson, 1985), amino acid analogs (Harms et al., 1982), or toxins from pathogens (Carlson, 1973; Gengenbach et al., 1977).

Horsch et al. (1987) recently demonstrated the value of the somatic cell genetic approach in the genetic engineering of plant resistance to the herbicide glyphosate. When isolated, as a result of a 20-fold amplification of the gene, a glyphosate-tolerant cell of petunia hybrid was shown to overproduce the enzyme (EPSP synthase) responsible for tolerance. A cDNA clone encoding the enzyme was isolated from a cDNA library of the tolerant cell line and used to transform herbicide-sensitive lines into tolerant cell lines.

Gamete culture can be used to generate haploids and doubled haploids for rapid development of homozygous breeding lines (Baenziger et al., 1984). Several new varieties of rice, tobacco, and barley have been developed with other culture techniques.

Protoplast fusion techniques are used to produce somatic hybrids by circumventing the usual sexual barriers among species and thus generating novel gene combinations (e.g., intergeneric combinations). Dudits and Praznovszky (1985) have shown that the production of asymmetric hybrids by fusion with irradiated protoplasts is an effective technique to create new gene combinations among distantly related plant species. The use of protoplasts to substitute or exchange cytoplasms to generate cytoplasmic male sterile (CMS) lines is of great practical value to plant breeders. This approach is a workable alternative to the generations of backcrossing usually required to convert a fertile line to a CMS line. Fusion techniques permit other genetic manipulation approaches to organelles (e.g., recombination); organelles are for the most part inaccessible for genetic improvement with conventional breeding methods.

Gene transfer technology offers the most precise manipulation of genetic traits. Most crop plants can now be efficiently transformed either through <u>Agrobacterium</u>-mediated gene transfer (Horsch et al., 1985), direct DNA transfer by uptake into protoplasts (Potrykus et al., 1985), or microinjection (Crossway et al., 1986). The practical utility of the molecular transfer of specific genes and their stable integration into the plant genome has been clearly demonstrated (Jaworski, see paper in this volume). This technology significantly extends the range of sources for genes beyond reach of conventional breeding and adds a new dimension to crop improvement strategies; these sources include viral genes (e.g., the tobacco mosaic virus coat protein) expressed in plants to confer resistance, bacterial genes (e.g., EPSP synthase) for herbicide tolerance (Comai et al., 1983), and insect genes (e.g., luciferase) for visual tracking and expression of transferred genes in situ (Ow et al., 1986). The ability to control the proper expression of introduced genes is critical to the usefulness of this technology. Several recent reports are encouraging in that regard. A seed storage protein gene of bean transferred to tobacco was shown to be properly expressed in a tissue-specific manner in tobacco seeds (Sengupta-Gopalan et al., 1985). Regulatory sequences of seed storage proteins from legumes and a nonseed protein gene cluster have been shown to operate correctly when transferred to tobacco. It is safe to assume that the routine introduction and expression of foreign genes in plants is close at hand. What is not so well advanced is knowledge of the genes that determine functional attributes in crop plants for food use.

Functional Attribute Genetics. There has been a serious neglect of research on the functional attributes of crops. By far the lion's share of both basic and applied research for crop improvement has been related to the production side: dealing with the agronomic traits, including disease and insect resistance, biochemical factors influencing yield, and stress and herbicide tolerance. This production-side or supply-side genetics affects supply, availability, and cost of raw materials. On the other hand, utilization-side or value-added genetics determines the processibility, nutrition, convenience, and quality of our raw materials and food products. The food industry has traditionally started with commodity raw materials, e.g., wheat, corn, and rice (Figure 3), and added value through processing technology to develop consumer products. We are now entering an era in the food industry when more emphasis will be placed on adding value further back in the food chain. Although this will be facilitated by the new genetic tools discussed above, it is severely limited by our current lack of understanding of functional attributes at the biochemical level. Also, many of the functional attribute traits are multigenic, which complicates genetic strategies for their improvement. Despite these limitations, we can expect to see a much greater emphasis on raw materials from crops that will be genetically tailored for the food processor and the consumer; the result will be "noncommodity" (Klausner, 1986), differentiated raw materials.

A clear demonstration of this has been the recent work with high-solids tomatoes. Increasing the solids content of tomatoes from 5% solids to a level of 6% solids has a value in the processed tomato industry worth $80-100 million per year. Several approaches are being pursued, but to date only the somaclonal variant line of DNA Plant Technology, called DNAP-9 (Certificate of Plant Variety Protection No. 8400146), has been released. DNAP-9 was derived from UC82B, a standard, open-pollinated processing variety, by regenerating plants from cultured tissues. Data submitted with the DNAP application filed in August 1984 indicate that the only principal difference is an increase in soluble solids of approximately 20% compared to that of UC82B. Although this appears to demonstrate the utility of the somaclonal variation approach, DNAP-9 may not be competitive with recently developed F_1 hybrids, which have higher yields and a roughly equivalent content of solids. DNAP and other companies are evaluating other somaclonal variant-derived hybrids. Molecular genetic approaches to increasing soluble solids in tomatoes have not demonstrated progress as yet.

The effect of mutant alleles in carbohydrate metabolism is well documented (Shannon and Garwood, 1984). With the genetic technologies being developed, it should be possible to specifically manipulate carbohydrate metabolism in cereal crops at the molecular level. Examples of food industry applications are improved texture and cooking properties of rice, enhanced sweetness and mouthfeel, e.g., creaminess of sweet corns, and antistaling characteristics of wheat flours for baked goods. From a somewhat different perspective, it should be possible to improve the texture of fruits and vegetables by inhibiting the expression of cellulase and pectinase during ripening (Wasserman et al., 1986).

Several strategies are being pursued to improve the essential amino acid balance of cereal grains and legume crops required in human and animal nutrition. Typically, cereals are deficient in lysine, and legumes are deficient in sulfur amino acids, methionine, and cysteine. Schaeffer (1986) and Hibberd et al. (1986) have reported the use of somatic cell genetics to select for cells that are resistant to amino acid analogs and that overproduce the deficient amino acids. Corn and rice plants regenerated from these cells have been shown to have higher levels of the specific amino acids in the grain. Molecular approaches are also making progress. Larkins (1987) reported that several laboratories are modifying seed storage protein genes by inserting specific sequences or making specific base substitutions to produce endogenous seed storage proteins containing higher levels of the limiting amino acids. Another approach involves either enhancing the expression of endogenous genes coding for nutritionally rich proteins or introducing seed storage protein genes from heterologous species to improve the amino acid balance (Rao and Singh, 1986). (The latter strategy is also being attempted for genes coding for the production of animal proteins, such as ovalbumin.) To date, none of these strategies has yielded an improved grain. In wheat, seed storage proteins control dough quality for baked goods, and these are amenable to similar genetic strategies.

Obviously, there are many other opportunities to improve the functional attributes of crops for the food industry. Several groups (Rattray, 1984; Sharp, 1986) are manipulating lipid biosynthesis to improve oil content and to modify triglyceride composition to enhance value (e.g., the production of coconut type oils in soybean or rapeseed). Unilever, Sime Darby, and the DNAP/United Fruit joint venture are currently establishing plantations of elite oil palm selections based on tissue culture cloning (Sharp, 1986). A 25 to 30% increase in yield of oil is predicted.

In plant biotechnology, there have been several very important advances that will affect our ability to modify functional attributes. The most important is the recent report of Ecker and Davis (1986) that antisense RNA (minus-strand RNA) inhibits specific gene expression in plants. Similar observations have been reported in bacterial and animal systems (Green et al., 1986). The practical importance of the antisense RNA approach to (in effect) generating instant mutant alleles is considerable. Not only can specific genes be blocked in a manner similar to mutations, but one antisense gene could also be used to block a multigene family. In addition, the antisense approach could be used to simulate a homozygous mutant allele, which would be of great value in polyploid species such as common bread wheat, which is hexaploid.

In plant cell technology, methods to transform cereal crops such as rice and corn (Fromm et al., 1986; Potrykus et al., 1985) and to regenerate plants from protoplasts (Abdullah et al., 1986) were recently reported. Soybeans, which have proven to be very resistant to cell culture manipulation, can also be regenerated (Collins et al., 1985). Thus, key techniques are now in place for most important food crops.

Production-Side Versus Utilization-Side Genetics

In this volume, Senator Albert Gore, Jr. (D-Tenn) has addressed the serious issue of the net effect of new applications of biotechnology on U.S. agriculture. Regarding the risks, he stated, "Given our record in dealing with agriculture, we are far more likely to accidentally drown ourselves in a sea of excess grain," and pointed out that we may further advance an age of intractable overproduction, promoting large-scale agribusiness farming at the expense of small farms. He asked, "Is the family farm about to be genetically altered out of existence?" And he concluded that with such an outcome, "Biotechnology will be a hollow victory for science or for society. . . ." These are valid points that reflect a perception shared by many of Senator Gore's colleagues who are involved in agricultural planning. This perception is based largely on the historically unbalanced agricultural research and development emphasis on production- or supply-side genetics (i.e., a focus on the production component of agriculture to achieve higher yields and lower costs of production). The majority of crop biotechnology is being applied to improvement of agronomic traits. This is especially true for both large corporations and small biotech companies, whose primary customer is the farmer.

However, in the food industry the recent increase in research in crop biotechnology is building momentum on the other side of the equation--utilization-side or value-added genetics. Here, research is oriented toward the end use of agricultural raw materials, with a focus on added value and higher return. There are great opportunities to extend the value-added food industry component back to the farm (Figure 3). Genetic improvement of specific crops for maximal return according to end use creates differentiated or noncommodity raw materials. The key to progress in this area will be research to develop a knowledge of the functionality of raw materials that is sufficient to be translated to genetic manipulation strategies. Companies that are successful in these efforts may generate an important new factor in technical leverage. The same may also be true at the international level.

Utilization-side or value-added genetics will bring about a certain degree of restructuring in agricultural practices (e.g., emphasizing contract crop production and raw material identity channels). Whether these changes will favorably affect the family farm is an important question to be addressed by agricultural economists. Regardless of which side of the crop improvement equation is pursued, the issue remains: Which specific genes or traits are to be selected as economically feasible targets?

Plant Cell Bioreactors

Thirty years ago, Routier and Nickell (1956) at Pfizer received a U.S. patent for the use of plant cell cultures for the industrial production of natural products. Since that time, considerable progress has been made in several areas: (1) in the number of plant species that can be grown in culture, (2) in the production of a wide array of secondary metabolites (Dougall, 1985), (3) in our understanding of the biochemical pathways involved and their regulation, and (4) in bioreactor design and culture protocols (Shuler and Hallsby, 1985). Despite these advances, there are only two commercial applications, and these are very high-value medicinals and cosmetic ingredients--shikonin (Tabata and Fujita, 1985) and ginsengoside (Ushiyama et al., 1986).

Long-range projections for inexpensive production of secondary metabolites, based on future technical developments, have been reported (Sahai and Knuth, 1985). However, the outlook for economical production of food ingredients by cell culture is not optimistic for the near term. This is due primarily to their relatively low value, low levels of production by cells, and the high cost of the plant cell bioreactor approach. The most recent estimate at the current state of the technology is roughly $3,000/kg (Drapeau et al., 1987). This appears to be a prime area for applying rDNA techniques to achieve the dramatic improvements required for commercial success.

ANIMAL BIOTECHNOLOGY

Most of the current applications of animal biotechnology relate to the production side (Evans and Hollaender, 1986); these include bovine growth hormone work, vaccine production, disease prevention, and embryo manipulations (sex selection, twinning, embryo storage, and transfer). Transgenic farm animals are still in the future. However, one area that relates to functional attributes for food is worth mentioning: genetic engineering of bovine milk proteins--the caseins. These are perhaps one of the most important and well-characterized groups of food proteins besides the seed storage proteins. Molecular work has advanced to the stage where systematic structure/function studies can be conducted on this class of proteins; this can lead to better understanding of food protein functionality.

Tom Richardson's group at the University of California, Davis, recently proposed a strategy involving protein engineering to change casein structure to improve function in food products (e.g., caseins with additional chymosin sites to accelerate the rate of texture development) (Kang et al., 1986). Commercial application of this strategy, however, must await progress in gene transfer and expression in animals.

CONCLUSIONS

Biotechnology Research in the Food Industry

The food industry is characteristically conservative in the amount it invests in research (typically, 1.5% or less of sales) and in its adoption of rapidly emerging areas of technology. As it now exists, biotechnology research is supported primarily by such typical power bases as DuPont and Monsanto and also by an increasing number of small research companies, the biotiques. Most of these small companies are quite skilled in their areas of expertise and are highly motivated, responsive, and productive. They represent the best of what we have come to recognize as the entrepreneurial spirit.

What we are seeing in food industry biotechnology is the effective use of research alliances between large food processors and the biotiques. This has allowed food companies to quickly attain critical mass in specialized areas of research and has served to accelerate developments in this area. Several of the examples used in this paper were the result of such alliances. This trend will continue. However, we are beginning to enter a new phase. As food companies become more familiar with the technology and begin to experience its success in the marketplace, we will see internalization of research skills and the full integration of biotechnology into the well-established food research disciplines.

Consolidation in the Food Industry

Acquisitions and mergers are common phenomena in the food industry. The result is the development of large corporations that are horizontally integrated across a broad spectrum of food sectors. As this occurs, along with the internationalization of biotechnology research skills, we will experience a strong movement toward vertical integration in the direction of our raw material base, which will position the "value-added cascade" to begin further back in the system, at the genetic level. This may represent the emergence of an important new fulcrum of competitive leverage in the food industry and may very well bring genetic biotechnology into its most productive arena.

REFERENCES

Abdullah, R., E.C. Cocking, and J.A. Thompson. 1986. Efficient plant regeneration from rice protoplasts through somatic embryogenesis. Bio/Technol. 4:1087-1090.

Arbige, M.V., P.R. Freund, S.C. Silver, and J.T. Zelko. 1986. Novel lipase for cheddar cheese flavor development. Food Technol. 40:91-96, 98.

Baenziger, P.S., D.T. Kudirka, G.W. Schaeffer, and M.D. Lazar. 1984. The significance of doubled haploid variation. Pp. 385-414 in J.P. Gustafson, ed. Genetic Manipulation in Plant Improvement. Plenum, New York.

Boyce, C.O.L. 1986. Novo's Handbook of Practical Biotechnology. Novo Industri A/S, Bagsvaerd, Denmark. 125 pp.

Carlson, P.S. 1973. Methionine sulfoximine-resistant mutants of tobacco. Science 180:1366-1368.

Casey, J.P. 1977. High fructose corn syrup: A case history of innovation. Staerke 29:196-204.

Charles Kline & Co. 1986. American market for enzymes expected to reach $260 million by 1990. Genet. Eng. News. 6:18.

Cocking, E.C. 1985. Somatic hybridization: Implications for agriculture. Pp. 101-113 in M. Zaitlin, P. Day, and A. Hollaender, eds. Biotechnology in Plant Science: Relevance to Agriculture in the Eighties. Academic Press, Orlando, Fla.

Coker, L.E., and K. Venkatasubramanian. 1985. Starch conversion processes. Pp. 777-788 in M. Moo-Young, H.W. Blanch, S. Drew, and D.I.C. Wang, eds. Comprehensive Biotechnology: The Practice of Biotechnology: Current Commodity Products, Vol. 3. Pergamon, Elmsford, N.Y.

Coleman, R.D., and M.P. McAlister. 1986. Plasmids containing a gene coding for a thermostable pullulanase and pullulanase-producing strains of Escherichia coli and Bacillus subtilis containing the plasmids. U.S. patent no. 4,612,287.

Collins, G.B., D.F. Hildebrand, P.A. Lazzeri, J.R. Myers, G. Benzion, M. Dahmer, and T.R. Adams. 1985. Cell culture systems for soybeans and clover with efficient plant regeneration via somatic embryogenesis. P. 26 in G.A. Galau, ed. Abstracts, First International Congress of Plant Molecular Biology. Organized by the International Society for Plant Molecular Biology, Oct. 27-Nov. 2, 1985, Savannah, Ga. Center for Continuing Education, University of Georgia, Athens, Ga.

Comai, L., L.C. Sen, and D.M. Stalker. 1983. An altered aroA gene product confers resistance to the herbicide glyphosate. Science 221:370-371.

Crossway, A., J.V. Oakes, J.M. Irvine, B. Ward, V.C. Knauf, and C.K. Skewmaker. 1986. Integration of foreign DNA following microinjection of tobacco mesophyll protoplasts. Mol. Gen. Genet. 202:179-185.

Dougall, D.K. 1985. Chemicals from plant cell cultures: Yields and variation. Pp. 179-190 in M. Zaitlin, P. Day, and A. Hollaender, eds. Biotechnology in Plant Science: Relevance to Agriculture in the Eighties. Academic Press, Orlando, Fla.

Drapeau, D., H.W. Blanch, and C.R. Wilke. 1987. Economic assessment of plant cell culture for the production of ajmalicine. Biotechnol. Bioeng. 30: 946-953.

Dudits, D., and T. Praznovszky. 1985. Intergenetic gene transfer by protoplasts fusion and uptake of isolated chromosomes. Pp. 115-127 in M. Zaitlin, P. Day, and A. Hollaender, eds. Biotechnology in Plant Science: Relevance to Agriculture in the Eighties. Academic Press, Orlando, Fla.

Earle, R.L. 1984. Food engineering and biotechnology. Food Technol. Aust. 36:498.

Ecker, J.R., and R.W. Davis. 1986. Inhibition of gene expression in plant cells by expression of antisense RNA. Proc. Natl. Acad. Sci. U.S.A. 83:5372-5376.

Evans, D.A., and W.R. Sharp. 1983. Single gene mutations in tomato plants regenerated from tissue culture. Science 221:949-951.

Evans, D.A., and W.R. Sharp. 1986. Applications of somaclonal variation. Bio/Technol. 4:528-532.

Evans, J.W., and A. Hollaender, eds. 1986. Genetic Engineering of Animals: An Agricultural Perspective. Plenum, New York. 336 pp.

Frey, N.M. 1984. Molecular biology in plant diagnostics. Pp. 427-439 in The World Biotech Report 1984, Vol. 2: USA. The Proceedings of Biotech 84, USA. Online, New York.

Fromm, M.E., L.P. Taylor, and V. Walbot. 1986. Stable transformation of maize after gene transfer by electroporation. Nature 319:791-793.

Gengenbach, B.G., C.E. Green, and C.M. Donovan. 1977. Inheritance of selected pathotoxin resistance in maize plants regenerated from cell cultures. Proc. Natl. Acad. Sci. U.S.A. 74:5113-5117.

Grant, J.D. 1986. Keys to effective biotechnology regulation: Scientific-based decisions and responsible industry action. Pp. 19-24 in A.T. Ganesan and J.A. Hoch, eds. Bacillus Molecular Genetics and Biotechnology Applications. Academic Press, Orlando, Fla.

Green, P.J., O. Pines, and M. Inouye. 1986. The role of antisense RNA in gene regulation. Annu. Rev. Biochem. 55:569-597.

Harlander, S.K., and T.P. Labuza, eds. 1986. Biotechnology in Food Processing. Noyes, Park Ridge, N.J. 349 pp.

Harms, C.T., J.J. Oertli, and J.M. Widholm. 1982. Characterization of amino acid analogue resistant somatic hybrid cell lines of Daucus carota L. Z. Pflanzenphysiol. 106:239-249.

Heyneker, H.L., D. Cullen, G.L. Gray, K.J. Hayenga, M.H. Lamsa, S. Norton, M.W. Rey, L.J. Wilson, and R.M. Berka. 1986. Cloning strategies in Aspergillus for enzyme production: Prochymosin as a model system. Pp. 145-149 in BIO EXPO 86: Proceedings of the American Commercial & Industrial Conference & Exposition in Biotechnology. Organized and presented by Cahners Exposition Group, April 29-May 1, 1986, Boston, Mass. Butterworth, Stoneham, Mass.

Hibberd, K.A., M. Barker, P.C. Anderson, and L. Linder. 1986. Selections for high tryptophan maize. P. 440 in D.A. Somers, B.G. Gengenbach, D.D. Biesboer, W.P. Hackett, and C.E. Green, eds. VI International Congress of Plant Tissue and Cell Culture, August 3-8, 1986, Abstracts. University of Minnesota, Minneapolis, Minn.

Horsch, R.B., J.E. Fry, N.L. Hoffmann, D. Eichholtz, S.G. Rogers, and R.T. Fraley. 1985. A simple and general method of transferring genes into plants. Science 227:1229-1231.

Horsch, R., R. Fraley, S. Rogers, J. Fry, H. Klee, D. Shah, S. McCormick, J. Niedermeyer, and N. Hoffmann. 1987. Agrobacterium-mediated transformation of plants. Pp. 317-329 in C.E. Green, D.A. Somers, W.P. Hackett, and D.D. Biesboer, eds. Plant Tissue and Cell Culture. Proceedings of the VI International Congress on Plant Tissue and Cell Culture held at the University of Minnesota, August 3-8, 1986. Alan R. Liss, New York.

Ishii, Y., M. Kanno, and M. Tamuri. 1981. Heat- and acid-stable alpha-amylase enzymes and processes for producing the same; culturing Bacillus, use to hydrolyze starch. U.S. patent no. 4,284,722.

Jarvis, B., and A.W. Holmes. 1982. Biotechnology in relation to the food industry. J. Chem. Technol. Biotechnol. 32:224-232.

Kang, Y., R. Jimenez-Flores, and T. Richardson. 1986. Casein genes and genetic engineering of the caseins. Pp. 95-111 in J.W. Evans and A. Hollaender, eds. Genetic Engineering of Animals: An Agricultural Perspective. Plenum, New York.

Kilara, A. 1982. Enzymes and their uses in the processed apple industry: A review. Process Biochem. 17:35-41.

Kirsop, B. 1985. Opportunities for biotechnology in food processing. Pp. 175-192 in G.E. Russell, ed. Biotechnology and Genetic Engineering Reviews, Vol. 3. Intercept, Dorset, England. Distributed by Scholium International, Great Neck, N.Y.

Klausner, A. 1986. Farmers can't succeed without agbiotech. Bio/Technol. 4:759.

Knorr, D.W., ed. 1987. Food Biotechnology. Marcel Dekker, New York. 625 pp.

Knorr, D., and A.J. Sinskey. 1985. Biotechnology in food production and processing. Science 229:1224-1229.

Larkin, P.J., S.A. Ryan, R.I.S. Brettell, and W.R. Scowcroft. 1984. Heritable somaclonal variation in wheat. Theor. Appl. Genet. 67:443-455.

Larkins, B.A. 1987. Modification of proteins encoded by seed storage protein genes. Pp. 163-167 in G. Bruening, J. Harada, T. Kosuge, and A. Hollaender, eds. Tailoring Genes for Crop Improvement: An Agricultural Perspective. Plenum, New York.

Lawrence, R.H., Jr. 1981. In vitro plant cloning systems. Environ. Exp. Bot. 21:289-300.

Lawrence, R.H., Jr., and P.E. Hill. 1982. Hybrids. U.S. patent no. 4,326,358.

Lawrence, R.H., Jr., and P.E. Hill. 1983. High purity hybrid cabbage seed production. U.S. patent no. 4,381,624.

Lin, Y.L. 1986. Genetic engineering and process development for production of food processing enzymes and additives. Food Technol. 40:104-112.

Lloyd, N.E., and R.O. Horwath. 1985. Biotechnology and the development of enzymes for the HFCS industry. Pp. 115-134 in BIO EXPO 85: World's Foremost Integrated Event on Biotechnology. Proceedings organized and presented by Cahners Exposition Group, May 14-16, 1985, Boston, Mass. Cahners Exposition Group, Stamford, Conn.

Lutz, J.D., J.R. Wong, J. Rowe, D.M. Tricoli, and R.H. Lawrence, Jr. 1985. Somatic embryogenesis for mass cloning of crop plants. Pp. 105-116 in R.R. Henke, K.W. Hughes, M.J. Constantin, and A. Hollaender, eds. Tissue Culture in Forestry and Agriculture. Plenum, New York.

McGuire, J. 1986. Cloning, expression, purification and testing of chymosin. Pp. 121-141 in BIO EXPO 86: Proceedings of the American Commercial & Industrial Conference & Exposition in Biotechnology. Organized and presented by Cahners Exposition Group, April 29-May 1, 1986, Boston, Mass. Butterworth, Stoneham, Mass.

Meade, J.H., T.J. White, S.P. Shoemaker, D.H. Gelfand, S. Chang, and M.A. Innis. 1987. Molecular cloning of carbohydrases for the food industry. Pp. 393-411 in D. Knorr, ed. Food Biotechnology. Marcel Dekker, New York.

Miller, O.K., and K.W. Hughes. 1980. Selection of paraquat-resistant variants of tobacco from cell cultures. In Vitro 16:1085-1091.

Moo-Young, M., H.W. Blanch, S. Drew, and D.I.C. Wang, eds. 1985. Comprehensive Biotechnology: The Practice of Biotechnology: Current Commodity Products, Vol. 3. Pergamon, Elmsford, N.Y. 1136 pp.

Nasrallah, J.B., and M.E. Nasrallah. 1985. The self-incompatibility locus of Brassica. Pp. 259-264 in M. Zaitlin, P. Day, and A. Hollaender, eds. Biotechnology in Plant Science: Relevance to Agriculture in the Eighties. Academic Press, Orlando, Fla.

Newsome, R.L. 1986. Sweeteners: Nutritive and non-nutritive. Food Technol. 40:195-206.

Ow, D.W., K.V. Wood, M. DeLuca, J.R. De Wet, D.R. Helinski, and S.H. Howell. 1986. Transient and stable expression of the firefly luciferase gene in plant cells and transgenic plants. Science 234:856-859.

Pitcher, W.H. 1986. Genetic modification of enzymes used in food processing. Food Technol. 40:62-63, 69.

Potrykus, I., M.W. Saul, J. Petruska, J. Paszkowski, and R.D. Shillito. 1985. Direct gene transfer to cells of a graminaceous monocot. Mol. Gen. Genet. 199:183-188.

Rao, A.S., and R. Singh. 1986. Improving grain protein quality by genetic engineering: Some biochemical considerations. Trends Biotechnol. 4:108-109.

Rattray, J.B.M. 1984. Biotechnology and the fats and oils industry: An overview. J. Am. Oil Chem. Soc. 61:1701-1712.

Redenbaugh, K., B.D. Paasch, J.W. Nichol, M.E. Kossler, P.R. Viss, and K.A. Walker. 1986. Somatic seeds: Encapsulation of asexual plant embryos. Bio/Technol. 4:797-801.

Rehm, H.J., and G. Reed, eds. 1983. Biotechnology, A Comprehensive Treatise in Eight Volumes: Food and Feed Production with Microorganisms, Vol. 5. VCH, Deerfield Beach, Fla. 473 pp.

Routier, J.B., and L.G. Nickell. 1956. Cultivation of plant tissue. U.S. patent no. 2,747,334.

Sahai, O., and M. Knuth. 1985. Commercializing plant tissue culture processes: Economics, problems, and prospects. Biotechnol. Prog. 1:1-9.

Schaeffer, G.W. 1986. Selection of rice, Oryza sativa, cells from inhibitory levels of lysine plus threonine and the characterization of the progeny. P. 439 in D.A. Somers, B.G. Gengenbach, D.D. Biesboer, W.P. Hackett, and C.E. Green, eds. VI International Congress of Plant Tissue and Cell Culture, August 3-8, 1986, Abstracts. University of Minnesota, Minneapolis, Minn.

Scowcroft, W.R., R.I.S. Brettell, P.A. Davies, P.J. Larkin, M.A. Pallotta, S.A. Ryan, and R. Appels. 1985. Somaclonal variation -- biology and agricultural impact. P. 4 in G.A. Galau, ed. Abstracts, First International Congress of Plant Molecular Biology. Organized by the International Society for Plant Molecular Biology, Oct. 27-Nov. 2, 1985, Savannah, Ga. Center for Continuing Education, University of Georgia, Athens, Ga.

Sengupta-Gopalan, C., N.A. Reichert, R.F. Barker, T.C. Hall, and J.D. Kemp. 1985. Developmentally regulated expression of the bean β-phaseolin gene in tobacco seed. Proc. Natl. Acad. Sci. U.S.A. 82:3320-3324.

Shaner, D.L., and P.C. Anderson. 1985. Mechanism of action of the imidazolinones and cell culture selection of tolerant maize. Pp. 287-299 in M. Zaitlin, P. Day, and A. Hollaender, eds. Biotechnology in Plant Science: Relevance to Agriculture in the Eighties. Academic Press, Orlando, Fla.

Shannon, J.C., and D.L. Garwood. 1984. Genetics and physiology of starch development. Pp. 25-86 in R.L. Whistler, J.N. BeMiller, and E.F. Paschall, eds. Starch: Chemistry and Technology, 2nd ed. Academic Press, Orlando, Fla.

Sharp, W.R., R.J. Whitaker, M.R. Sondahl, D.A. Evans, J.E. Bravo, J.F. Marsden, R.J. Orton, and L.C.S. Ramos. 1986. Opportunities for biotechnology in the development of new edible vegetable oil products. J. Am. Oil Chem. Soc. 63:594-595, 598-600.

Shuler, M.L., and G.A. Hallsby. 1985. Bioreactor considerations for chemical production from plant cell cultures. Pp. 191-205 in M. Zaitlin, P. Day, and A. Hollaender, eds. Biotechnology in Plant Science: Relevance to Agriculture in the Eighties. Academic Press, Orlando, Fla.

Snow, R. 1985. Genetic engineering of a yeast strain for malolactic fermentation of wine. Food Technol. 39:96, 98-101, 109.

Tabata, M., and Y. Fujita. 1985. Production of shikonin by plant cell cultures. Pp. 207-218 in M. Zaitlin, P. Day, and A. Hollaender, eds. Biotechnology in Plant Science: Relevance to Agriculture in the Eighties. Academic Press, Orlando, Fla.

Ushiyama, K., H. Oda, and Y. Miyamoto. 1986. Large scale tissue culture of Panax ginseng root. P. 252 in D.A. Somers, B.G. Gengenbach, D.D. Biesboer, W.P. Hackett, and C.E. Green, eds. VI International Congress of Plant Tissue and Cell Culture, August 3-8, 1986, Abstracts. University of Minnesota, Minneapolis, Minn.

Wasserman, B.P., L.L. Eiberger, and K.J. McCarthy. 1986. Biotechnological approaches for controlled cell wall glucan biosynthesis in fruits and vegetables. Food Technol. 40:90-93, 96-98.

Williams, S.A., R.A. Hodges, T.L. Strike, R. Snow, and R.E. Kunkee. 1984. Cloning the gene for the malolactic fermentation of wine from Lactobacillus delbrueckii in Escherichia coli and yeasts. Appl. Environ. Microbiol. 47:288-293.

Yocum, R.R. 1986. Genetic engineering of industrial yeasts. Pp. 171-180 in BIO EXPO 86: Proceedings of the American Commercial & Industrial Conference & Exposition in Biotechnology. Organized and presented by Cahners Exposition Group, April 29-May 1, 1986, Boston, Mass. Butterworth, Stoneham, Mass.

II

BIOTECHNOLOGY: FOOD SAFETY AND NEW ROLES FOR TRADITIONAL INSTITUTIONS

POTENTIAL FOOD SAFETY PROBLEMS RELATED TO NEW USES OF BIOTECHNOLOGY

Jack Doyle

In a recent edition of Business Week, it was reported that a 35-year-old plant geneticist named Brent Tisserat, working for the U.S. Department of Agriculture in a basement laboratory in Pasadena, California, produced orange juice from test-tube cultures of orange cells. In this Pasadena laboratory, the juice-sac cells from oranges are surgically removed from mature fruit and placed in a tissue culture medium, where they remain alive for as long as 8 months, approaching the size of cells found in tree-ripened fruit. The juice that has been extracted from the orange cells in this cell-culture system is "chemically similar to what is squeezed from tree-grown fruit" (Flynn, 1986). Tisserat has also succeeded in culturing juice-producing vesicles from lemons and citrons. In addition to these citrus cultures, there are also thousands of miniature spinach, carrot, and other crops being grown in test tubes in Tisserat's laboratory.

Tisserat's tissue culture work has attracted the attention of the citrus industry and has been studied by Coca-Cola officials from the company's Minute Maid subsidiary. Allen V. Clark, manager of citrus research and development for Coca-Cola Company Foods, which markets Minute Maid orange juice, says he is awed by Tisserat's accomplishment. In the near term, culturing citrus-juice sacs in the laboratory could advance trait selection work in the nurseries and speed up varietal development.

Dan A. Kimball, director of research for California's Citrus Producers, Inc., says that the culturing of citrus juice sacs could help "standardize the entire citrus-juice industry." Others are more sanguine about the prospect of laboratory-produced juice, saying that it may take 15 to 25 years before it is commercially feasible on a large scale (Flynn, 1986).

Nevertheless, such work is moving forward, and others are culturing cocoa and cotton cells in the laboratory (Associated Press, 1985) and cloning all sorts of plants and tree crops for food, fiber, and oil. These developments will change the way food is produced and, conceivably, the way food looks, tastes, and provides nutrients.

BIOTECHNOLOGY AND THE PRODUCTION COMMAND IN AGRICULTURE

Biotechnology is revolutionary for agriculture and the food system, because it places control over food production *in the genes*. Food production, of course, has always been empowered by genes, but we haven't been able to see them, precisely select them, or move them across traditional species barriers. Now we can. And day by day we are learning which traits in crops and livestock are controlled by individual genes, how to turn those genes on and off, how to splice them into the organisms, and how to amplify gene products.

So first, we have an awesome new technology that operates at the *genetic level* of the food system--the most fundamental level of food characterization. This means that the production and quality commands in the food system begin with the genes and, most importantly, with those who hold the genes and wield the new genetic technologies.

Second, coupled with the new genetic technologies is the *legal* power to own genes. Those who have been following the legal developments in the biological realm over the last 6 years or so know that genes can now be patented, as can certain techniques used in genetic manipulation (U.S. Supreme Court, 1980). This means that an inventor or commercial interest can have a property right in genetic material. In economic terms, that means having an exclusive marketing right--a limited monopoly for 17 years or more--on genetic "inventions" and certain genetic techniques.

Third, in the realm of food and agriculture, there are quite obviously a lot of genes. There are genes that control yield in corn, stalk strength in barley, protein levels in wheat, and the efficiency of photosynthesis in soybeans. In livestock, there are genes that have to do with fat content, lactation rates, feed-to-meat conversion rates, growth, and disease resistance.

In fact, it is possible to imagine a classification system of sought-after traits, including, for example, <u>agronomic</u> <u>traits</u> such as those for higher yield or harvestability in crop production; <u>food-processing</u> <u>traits</u> such as those governing less water or more solids in certain fruits and vegetables; <u>food quality traits</u> such as those controlling higher protein levels in crops or lower fat content in livestock; and traits pursued for their <u>public health</u> or <u>environmental benefits</u> such as genetic alterations to crops and livestock that would dispense with the need to use pesticides or antibiotics in the agricultural environment. But which traits will be pursued first? Can all traits be pursued simultaneously? And what does this mean for food quality and food safety?

FOOD QUALITY AND FOOD SAFETY

Biotechnology in agricultural production and food processing may affect the quality and safety of food in several direct and indirect ways: (1) by displacing or altering the genes that control the nutritional constituents of food crops and livestock; (2) by altering the genes that affect the levels of naturally occurring toxins in food crops, livestock, or fish; and (3) by extending certain agricultural production practices, such as the use of pesticides, that lead to chemical residues in food and water.

Biotechnology and the Genes of Nutrition

Today, there is much talk about the nutritional improvement of crops with the help of biotechnology and genetic engineering.

• As stated by the Kellogg Company in 1981, "Through the advances afforded by genetic engineering, grains will become more widely accepted because of improvements in taste, texture, form, and total nutritional profile" (Kellogg Co., 1981, p. 2).

• In a brochure entitled "Genetic Engineering: A Natural Science," the Monsanto Company lists "food plants with enhanced nutritional value" as one of the possible results of biotechnological research now under way (Monsanto Co., 1984, p. 11). Writing in the November 1985 issue of Science '85, Monsanto executive Howard Schneiderman explained that certain tropical root crops, such as cassava and taro, could be genetically engineered for more protein and less cyanide (Schneiderman, 1985).

• The Rockefeller Foundation, in its continuing commitment to the genetics of rice improvement, has made major research grants to develop through genetic engineering a variety of yellow rice that would produce carotene in the grain to help fight vitamin A deficiency in developing countries where diets consist primarily of rice (Rockefeller Foundation, 1985).

• In the United States, several corporate and university laboratories are focusing on the genetics of nutrition. For example, Phytogen, a biotechnology subsidiary of J.G. Boswell Co., one of the nation's largest farms, is attempting to "increase the nutritional quality of the protein" in the russett Burbank potato with recombinant DNA techniques (Anderson, 1984, p. 6).

• At the University of California, Los Angeles (UCLA), researchers have been working to unearth the genetic mechanisms governing the seed storage protein in soybeans and other crops, which are deficient in some amino acids essential to human nutrition.

Some nutritionists are opposed to genetic engineering for nutritional improvement, fearing that such tampering with the genes of nutrition might cause a great fluctuation in nutrient levels in commercial cultivars and create a kind of nutritional havoc within the national food system. In fact, some nutritionists would rather we be vigilant about nutritional erosion that might be taking place in raw food crops due to genetic engineering for other purposes, e.g., to obtain certain food processing traits or to achieve higher crop yields. In fact, do we really know what is happening to the nutritional integrity of food crops that are being altered for these purposes?

We know from experience in classical plant breeding that some tomato varieties bred for mechanical harvesting in California during the late 1960s suffered a 15% reduction in vitamin C content (Spiher, 1975). In this case, the genes that were desirable for mechanical harvesting were inversely related to those needed for maintaining high vitamin C levels.

Similarly, in Europe, the nutrient levels of some potato varieties have been altered because of farm production and food processing demands. In the United Kingdom, for example, the nutrient levels of some potato varieties are considerably lower than those stated in the U.K. Food Composition Tables--namely, 50% lower in riboflavin and niacin, 40% lower in potassium, and 20 to 30% lower in iron, copper, and zinc. On the other hand, thiamine and folic acid in some of these potato varieties were 2 to 3 times higher (Gormley et al., 1986).

So, the important questions here are: What will be improved? What does "improve" mean? And who will make those decisions?

INTEGRATING BACKWARD

In a speech before the Industrial Biotechnology Association in October 1986 in San Francisco, Roger Salquist, Chief Executive Officer of the biotechnology company Calgene, asked his audience what names were brought to mind in association with agricultural biotechnology. "It's not necessarily the farmers," he said. "It's the Campbell Soup companies, the Kraft Food Company, the R.J. Reynolds Company" (Salquist, 1986, p. 2). In his view, these are the interests that are investing in and will commercialize biotechnology in agriculture.

According to Salquist, the major processing companies that used to buy their agricultural crops on the open commodity markets are going to stake out a proprietary interest in those crops because they can command the genes in those crops for specific ends:

> Look at the major processors now; they all have their own breeding programs. In essence, they're not just going out and buying tomatoes on the market; they're creating their own tomatoes to have the specific traits they want to have for higher value. And, you're going to see that across the board--from brewing companies, to food companies, to tobacco companies. They're engineering products and integrating backwards (Salquist, 1986, p. 5).

Indeed, the Congressional Office of Technology Assessment is inclined to agree with Salquist on this last point, noting in its March 1986 report "Technology, Public Policy, and the Changing Structure of American Agriculture" that contracting and vertical integration in agriculture and food production are likely to increase with advances in biotechnology because of the control it offers over the genetic elements of production (U.S. Congress, Office of Technology Assessment, 1985).

BIOTECHNOLOGY AND THE FOOD PROCESSING INDUSTRY

Food processing companies have been among some of the earliest and, recently, most aggressive investors in biotechnology:

- In March 1982, the Campbell Soup Company began a contractual relationship with DNA Plant Technology Corporation to conduct research to determine the genetic basis for improving the solids content of tomatoes (Morris, 1982). Heinz followed suit in December of that year in a research contract with the Atlantic Richfield Company's Plant Cell Research Institute. Every 1% increase in the solids content of tomatoes is worth about $80 million annually in processing savings (L. William Teweles & Co., 1983).

- In June 1982, the Kellogg Company invested $10 million in Agrigenetics, an agricultural biotechnology company now owned by Lubrizol. At the time of Kellogg's investment in Agrigenetics, Kellogg chairman William

LaMothe said that it give his company access to "a field becoming increasingly important to Kellogg's long-term future" (Anonymous, 1982, p. 8). Kellogg and Agrigenetics also agreed to conduct joint research on ways to increase the protein content of cereal grains, to arrest mold resistance in corn, and to develop new corn lines capable of producing higher yields of cornstarch.

- American Home Products is trying to develop a popcorn that is edible without salt and butter by genetically altering corn plants to produce a more flavorful kernel (Lewis, 1986).

- General Foods has contracted with investigators to seek a low-caffeine coffee bean to reduce its decaffeination costs (Lewis, 1986).

- Hershey Foods is seeking new varieties of cocoa trees that will produce a bean with lower levels of the naturally occurring bitter flavors that must now be masked during processing (Lewis, 1986).

- Nestlé is attempting to develop a genetic engineering system for soybeans in conjunction with Calgene, Inc., a California biotechnology company (Calgene, Inc., 1986).

- Kraft, Inc., is producing and marketing a new line of carrot and celery vegetable snacks with the tradename VegiSnax. These vegetable products are developed in a tissue culture process known as somaclonal variation, in which natural genetic variation produces mutants that can be selected for particular characteristics. VegiSnax have already been test-marketed as 100% natural, ready-to-eat, low-calorie vegetable sticks, said to be crisper, crunchier, and sweeter than those available in existing varieties. They will be sold in snack-size packages and priced to compete with products such as potato chips. VegiSnax also have one other important feature: added shelf life. They will retain their genetically selected crispness and crunch for up to 2 weeks (DNA Plant Technology Corp., 1985).

While all this work is going on in the food processing industry, who is watching out for inadvertant changes in the nutritional integrity of food crops or livestock?

NATURALLY OCCURRING TOXICANTS

A second food safety issue involving the use of biotechnology and genetic engineering in food crops concerns naturally occurring toxins. Through bioengineering techniques, it may be possible to inadvertently turn on or magnify the background levels of certain naturally occurring toxins found in many food crops. Alternatively, it might also be possible, through the introduction or addition of genes from other plant species, to inadvertently introduce new toxins into agricultural crops.

In 1967, the U.S. Department of Agriculture (USDA) released a new potato variety named Lenape, which the agency believed to be potentially valuable for making potato chips. In fact, its formal press release on the variety carried the following headline: "A New Potato Unusually High in Solids and Chipping Qualities." In the USDA announcement, the Wise Potato Chip Company of Pennsylvania was singled out by name for helping in evaluating and testing the Lenape. Within the next year or so, the variety was being planted for seed potatoes in the United States and Canada. But in 1969, two Canadians discovered quite by accident (one of them got sick after eating some Lenapes) that this particular variety had very high levels of glycoalkaloids--naturally occurring substances found in potatoes, eggplants, peppers, and tomatoes that at high concentrations can cause severe illness (Zitnak and Johnston, 1970). In a few instances in Europe, high glycoalkaloid concentrations in potatoes have been associated with intestinal disorders and even death of humans and livestock (Doyle, 1985a).

After a round of controversy and some resistance to pulling the variety off the market, the USDA and the Pennsylvania Agricultural Experiment Station issued a joint statement in February 1970 withdrawing the Lenape from further agricultural use. In its announcement, USDA noted that the Lenape was found to contain approximately twice the level of glycoalkaloids carried by commercial varieties of potatoes. "This variety is no longer recommended for planting," said the announcement, "and no basic seed stocks will be released in the future." In addition, USDA warned that "Lenape variety potatoes are not suited for boiling or baking." The consumption of whole Lenape potatoes prepared this way, explained USDA, "might produce discomfort or even illness." It was this possibility, said the agency in its announcement, that caused it to withdraw the variety (USDA, 1970, p. 1).

Today, of course, we know that there are innumerable other examples of naturally occurring toxins in agricultural food crops, some of which are known carcinogens or mutagens. Rhubarb, spinach, cottonseed, black pepper, beets, celery, figs, parsley, parsnips, fava beans, and mustard seed are but a few of the crops that harbor some identified naturally occurring toxins of one kind or another (Ames, 1983). Although little is known about naturally occurring toxins in plants, most of the identified compounds are believed to be harmless at low levels, but could be a problem if elevated to higher levels, especially in raw food crops.

As the Lenape potato incident makes plain, even with classical genetics we have been able to increase the levels of some naturally occurring toxins inadvertently. Now, with the faster pace of biotechnology and gene splicing and the ability to cross species barriers and move exotic germplasm and genes into commercial cultivars, we might find ourselves changing toxin levels, introducing totally new ones, or creating a secondary situation that invites the creation of a toxin.

Bruce Ames, chairman of the Department of Biochemistry at the University of California, Berkeley, noted that plant breeders have developed a new strain of glandless cotton with low levels of gossypol, a naturally occurring toxin in cottonseed. Gossypol is a suspected carcinogen and is reported to cause abnormal sperm and male sterility in rats and humans. However, seeds from the low-gossypol cotton variety are more susceptible to attack by the fungus that produces the potent carcinogen aflatoxin (Ames, 1983).

Similarly, plant breeders are now moving genes from a species of poisonous lettuce (Lactuca virosa) to commercial varieties of lettuce to increase insect resistance. The poisonous lettuce variety contains substances shown to be mutagenic (Ames, 1983).

As with nutritional alteration, the questions again are: Do we know what is being changed? And who is monitoring crops for such changes?

BIOTECHNOLOGY AND CHEMICAL RESIDUES IN THE FOOD SYSTEM

A third area of concern is how biotechnology might change the use of chemicals in agriculture. Biotechnology offers some promise for reducing or eliminating the use of pesticides and synthetic fertilizers in the environment, and this should reduce the occurrence of chemical residues in food and water. Potential breakthroughs, such as nitrogen-fixing cereal crops or crops genetically engineered with more durable forms of resistance to diseases and insects, promise to move us away from the pesticide era.

Recently, companies such as Monsanto and Rohm & Haas have made some advances in such work: Monsanto with tobacco-mosaic virus restistance in tomatoes and tobacco, and Rohm & Haas in moving the insect toxin gene from the bacterium <u>Bacillus thuringiensis</u> into a model tobacco plant (Schmeck, 1986). In addition, a number of companies and researchers are interested in genetically engineered microbial pesticides, which may also displace chemical pesticides. Yet these genetically altered organisms pose a different, and in many cases, unknown set of ecological risks (Alexander, 1985).

Despite the applications of biotechnology that may eventually help reduce the load of toxic agricultural chemicals in the environment, other applications may <u>extend</u> the pesticide era and invite further capital investment in pesticide production. One such area is the work now being conducted to make crops resistant to chemicals, not to pests. And here I'm referring to herbicide resistance--that is, giving crops the genes to tolerate or resist herbicides that formerly killed or damaged them. At least 25 companies, as well as a number of university and USDA researchers, are working to make a number of major crops, including corn, wheat, cotton, and soybeans, genetically resistant to one or more herbicides (Doyle, 1985b).

This past July, Ciba-Geigy conducted the first USDA-approved field test of atrazine-resistant tobacco plants in North Carolina (Ciba-Geigy Corp., 1986a,b). Genetic resistance in crops to at least a dozen other herbicides is also being sought. This application of biotechnology is troubling from a public health standpoint, since many herbicides are now being found in drinking water and underground water supplies, and a number have been identified as potential carcinogens (Doyle, 1985b, 1986).

In addition to the work on herbicide resistance, there is research on the use of chemical plant growth regulators to turn on or turn off the genes in crops to do one or more specific things during growth. If commercialized, both lines of research will extend the pesticide era in agriculture rather than end it and are likely to increase public exposure to pesticides (Doyle, 1986).

THE CAPITALIZATION OF COMMERCIALLY FAVORED GENES

It is becoming increasingly clear from the activities of the last several years that major companies with interests in the input side of agriculture (i.e, in seed, pesticides, and fertilizers) such as Monsanto and Ciba-Geigy, as well as those with interests in processing, handling, and selling food products, such as General Foods and Campbell have all begun to make sizeable capital investments in genetics to achieve certain ends. In some cases, the investments are being made in particular genes, such as herbicide-resistant genes or high-solids tomato genes. In other cases, the entire genome of a new crop variety or particular livestock breed has been capitalized into the food system.

The Adolph Coors Company has contracts with some 2,500 farmers who grow a Coors-owned barley variety named Moravian III. This variety is grown over several hundred thousand acres in Colorado, Wyoming, and Montana. Del Monte and Green Giant specify certain vegetable varieties in contracts they have with Wisconsin vegetable growers. The Quaker Oats Company publishes a recommended list of white corn hybrids for its contract farmers in Iowa, Kansas, Missouri, the Ohio Valley, and in the Southeast (Doyle, 1985a).

The McDonald's Corporation has built a worldwide french-fry empire on the genes of the russet Burbank potato (Cox, 1982). In each of these examples, factories have been calibrated around the performance of a certain specific variety or a particular set of genes. And in the future, we're going to see more of this kind of thing, not less.

Not only do these examples raise questions about genetic uniformity and the agricultural vulnerability that goes with it, but also questions about the difficulty of reversing the use of products with large capital investments behind them. If the predominant capital interests are wrapped up in the genes of the russet Burbank potato, for example, how much chance does another variety really have? Similarly, if food processing genes are the primary focus of the food processing industry and the biotechnology companies seeking their attention, what happens when a nutritional trait lies in the way of the sought-after food processing trait? And who's to know when that happens? Who makes the decisions in those cases?

The point here is that capital momentum in biotechnology research, even at this very early stage, could determine what traits are pursued, which ones remain intact, and which ones are not pursued. And in this process, the public interest in food safety and food quality may not be adequately represented by the operation of the market. The question then becomes one of regulation. But is the current regulatory apparatus adequate for ensuring that all genetically altered crops and livestock will not suffer nutritional fluctuations or toxicant changes?

BIOTECHNOLOGY AND FOOD SAFETY REGULATION

In December 1970, the U.S. Food and Drug Administration (FDA) proposed that "foods that have had a significant alteration of composition by breeding or selection" be included for review and regulation under the review process for food additives Generally Recognized as Safe (GRAS) (FDA, 1970, p. 18624). The intent of this proposal was to review raw food crops with changes in naturally occurring toxicants or nutritional constituents as a result of breeding. It was the first time that FDA had ever attempted to regulate raw agricultural crops rather than finished products made from crops. The FDA regulation became final on June 1971 and remains on the books today. Yet no guidelines exist, and it is unclear just how FDA has handled this regulation since 1971.

One query from the Environmental Policy Institute to FDA regarding the GRAS regulation in 1984 yielded a limited response from Sanford Miller, then Director of FDA's Center for Food Safety and Applied Nutrition. Miller indicated that the regulation was still operative; that the agency had dealt with many inquiries about new varieties on a case-by-case basis, but that no list of such inquiries was available; and that no enforcement actions on this regulation were ever taken by the agency. Miller also noted that livestock were not excluded from the regulation, although USDA would have primary responsibility. He also added that "FDA has never established a mandatory monitoring program for the purpose of checking the level of nutrients or toxicants in new varieties of food substances" (Doyle, 1985a, p. 153). He indicated, however, that potatoes were monitored on a voluntary basis, but that this was handled through USDA.

One of the reasons why to this day the FDA plant breeding regulation does not have guidelines is the lack of data on nutrient levels and naturally occurring toxins.

THE 1973 NATIONAL RESEARCH COUNCIL REPORT ON GENETIC ALTERATIONS IN FOOD AND FEED CROPS

In August 1973, the eight-member National Research Council Task Force on Genetic Alterations in Food and Feed Crops submitted a short report to the Board on Agriculture and the Food and Nutrition Board. In this report, Task Force chairman Warren H. Gableman of the University of Wisconsin noted, "The Task Force feels strongly that this is an area of critical national concern. We sincerely hope the recommendations submitted herewith can be implemented without delay" (Gabelman et al., 1973, cover page).

Although the Task Force recommendations were not acted upon because of the lack of funds to undertake a larger study and because the focus of the report was plant breeding and not biotechnology, its observations and findings are nonetheless quite salient to our situation today. What follows are some excerpts from the report.

First, a general observation from the report:

> If the world's steadily increasing demand for food is to be met, the plant breeder must be

given opportunity to apply all the tools available to him to enhance productivity, pest resistance, nutritional quality and desirable processing characteristics while preventing increases in toxicants and maintaining product acceptability. Wherever possible, federal regulations should encourage rather than hamper the breeder in his efforts (p. 1).

On lack of data pertaining to nutritive qualities:

In reference information, e.g., USDA Handbook 8, data on nutritive value tend to be limited to species, and little information is provided either on differences among various cultivars of a species, or on the extent to which differences among species are genetic and (or) environmental in origin. Information from "The New Crops Branch" of the USDA seldom documents nutritional value or toxic components of any of their germ plasm resources (p. 2).

Elsewhere in the report, the Task Force notes, "At present there are inadequate data to serve as reference standards by plant breeders on the nutritional value of food and feed supplies" (p. 3). And there are references made to inadequate data collection and poor methodologies for evaluating nutrients:

Even when samples are properly characterized there are serious methodological problems in the determination of some of the major nutrients. . . . There are also serious methodological problems associated with the determination of the biological availability or activity of iron, zinc, and other micro-nutrients, folic acid, carotenoids as precursors of vitamin A and a number of other nutrients where their availability can be influenced by either the presence or absence of specific plant constituents (p. 4).

On the matter of biological assays for use in plant breeding, the Task Force noted, "Microassays and ultramicroassays must be developed for screening rapidly large numbers of very small samples so that reliable guides to the biological availability of specific nutrients will be provided" (p. 4).

On the topic of nutritional goals, the report notes:

> It is desirable to avoid a significant decrease of those specific nutrients in plants recognized as good sources of these nutrients. Where plants are not a significant source of specific nutrients, there is little need for concern with variations in content. Specific crops for which an improvement in one or more selected nutrients would be of practical nutritional significance should be identified and authoritative recommendations made to plant breeders to achieve increases in these nutrients whenever feasible, while maintaining adequate acceptability of the food.
>
> [Until] now in plant breeding programs the nutritional goals have either been ignored or are secondary to yield and pest resistance. The relevant nutritional characteristics of new varieties should in the future be identified prior to their commercial introduction. Nutritional characteristics could become on a par with yield and pest resistance. This would encourage the application of appropriate regulatory standards to prevent progressive depletion of the nutritional quality of the national supply of food and feed and encourage its improvement (p. 6).

On the topic of toxins in plants, the Task Force was equally critical of the lack of data and policy. "For the guidance of plant breeders there is a critical need to develop improved methods for the measurement of toxicants in plants and for the accumulation of data on their occurrence." It explained, "It would be sound policy . . . to avoid significant increases in the level of toxicants in the crops which are major components of the diets of man or of domestic and farm animals" (pp. 9-10). And guidelines were recommended:

> Guidelines for plant breeders should be developed . . . for those crops known to have naturally occurring toxicants of potential significance in terms of their use patterns. . . .

> For naturally occurring compounds which are known to be a problem, analytical data should be obtained prior to the release of any new cultivar known to be a source of these products. For those toxicants which represent a problem or limitation to the use of current cultivars, plant breeders should be encouraged to explore their reduction through genetic means (p. 10).

Earlier in the report, the Task Force explained:

> <u>There is an urgent need</u> for expert groups competent in nutrition and in toxicology <u>to develop guidelines which will indicate to plant breeders those changes in chemical composition of plants used for food or feed which are desirable, undesirable or of no practical significance.</u> These guidelines will need to be developed for each of the major food and feed crops since the relative biological significance of chemical changes will vary from one to another. For some nutrients, and many potentially toxic substances, there is insufficient information available to establish reliable goals or limits and analytical methods are often inadequate for their implementation (p. 5).

Unfortunately, the situation hasn't changed much in any of these data or analytical areas since this report was filed. But with biotechnology now upon us, the research called for by the 1973 Task Force is even <u>more urgent</u> than it was 14 years ago. Accordingly, I would urge the Academy to revisit this issue very soon, and consider launching a major review in this area.

BIOTECHNOLOGY, CONSUMERS, AND THE FOOD QUALITY MOVEMENT

How will consumers react to the changes in agriculture and food processing that will soon arrive with biotechnology? It is clear that in the last 6 years or so, there has been growing consumer concern over food safety and increasing interest in food quality. In a January 1984 consumer survey conducted by the Food Marketing Institute, 77% of those polled expressed concern over pesticide and herbicide residues in food, indicating the problem to be a "serious hazard" (Hammonds, 1985). Such concerns over food safety have also begun to penetrate the business community.

On November 7, 1986, in the Wall Street Journal, for example, it was reported that the H.J. Heinz Company was planning to restrict the purchase of crops used in the manufacture of baby foods that had been treated with certain pesticides. Heinz listed 12 chemicals: alachlor, aldicarb, captan, captafol, carbofuran, carbon tetrachloride, cyanazine, daminozide, dinocap, ethylene oxide, linuron, and triphenyltin hydroxide (TPTH). Heinz told farmers that it would probably test crops for the absence of these chemicals--all of which are still legal but under review by the Environmental Protection Agency (EPA) as possible health hazards (Meier, 1986).

On July 17, 1986, Safeway Stores, Inc., the nation's largest grocery chain, announced that it would stop buying apples treated with the chemical growth regulator Alar, despite EPA's decision in January to allow its use while further studies are done. In addition, the State of Maine proposed a nondetectable standard for daminozide, and the Commonwealth of Massachusetts has enacted regulation to reduce Alar in baby foods and heat-processed foods to a nondetectable level by 1988 (Anonymous, 1986).

In May 1986, United Farmworkers leader Cesar Chavez sent out a mass mailing appeal to Americans nationwide, announcing a new grape boycott aimed at eliminating five pesticides that endanger the health of farmworkers. In his appeal, Chavez asked consumers not to buy fresh California table grapes until growers agree to ban the five most dangerous pesticides used in grape production-- captan, dinoseb, parathion, phosdrin, and methyl bromide (Chavez, 1986).

Also in May 1986, the Center for Science in the Public Interest began a national campaign called "Americans for Safe Food." Included was a five-point plan of action urging consumers to:

- organize a grassroots movement of citizens who are concerned about the safety of the food supply;

- encourage widespread availability of contaminant-free foods;

- fight for laws that require disclosure of pesticides, drugs, and other chemicals used in the production of foods;

- demand a ban on pesticides and animal drugs known to pose a serious risk to consumers; and

- press for national standards for "organic," "natural," and "pesticide-free" foods (Center for Science in the Public Interest, 1986).

In Europe, meanwhile, there is also a growing concern over food safety, as expressed in the recent ban on animal growth hormones (Dixon, 1986).

In addition to the actions being taken on pesticides, increasing scientific attention has been focused on the association between diet and cancer and between diet and heart disease. In June 1982, the National Academy of Science released the report <u>Diet, Nutrition, and Cancer,</u> which emphasized the importance of eating fruits and vegetables high in vitamins C and A and noted that vegetables in the cabbage family contain natural cancer-inhibiting substances (NRC, 1982).

In February 1984, the American Cancer Society launched a national campaign for an anticancer diet, complete with dietary guidelines suggesting a reduction of total fat intake and an increase in the consumption of whole-grain cereals, fruits, and vegetables (Russell, 1984). In May 1984, the American Heart Association offered its dietary plan to help Americans lower their blood fat levels, including recommendations for eating less red meat and more fruits and vegetables (Brody, 1984).

The national concern about diet, food safety, and food quality has not been lost on the new biotechnology companies. One such company is DNA Plant Technology Corporation of New Jersey, which offered the following statement in a March 1986 public offering prospectus distributed on Wall Street:

> The Company believes that changing lifestyles and a growing consciousness of the importance

of proper nutrition for overall health and
fitness are changing eating habits in the
United States and other developed countries.
As people have become increasingly aware of the
risks associated with too much cholesterol,
sodium, fat, and calories in the diet, demand
for 100% natural, healthful foods has
increased. At the same time, the Company
believes that changes in the work environment
and family patterns have accelerated the
public's need for convenience in eating (DNA
Plant Technology Corp., 1986, p. 15).

Armed with this view of consumer needs, the company developed VegiSnax, a bioengineered snack food described earlier. Whatever the nutritional worth of this product may be, VegiSnax is also being billed as an example of how biotechnology might help food processors sell fruits and vegetables. "Once food processors can control the charaterisitics of the fruits and vegetables they market," explains Adweek, "they can slap brands on them, as Kraft is doing with VegiSnax" (Shields, 1985, p. 4).

In May 1986 at a meeting of stockholders, Richard Laster, president and CEO of DNA Plant Technology, said that he believes agricultural biotechnology creates an "opportunity to do to the quality . . . of the plant-based products we eat, what the first green revolution a few decades ago did to the quantity of food we have available" (Laster, 1986, p. 3). We certainly hope that turns out to be the case.

It is true, of course, that there is a lot of consumer and environmental agitation for safer food, as well as mounting scientific evidence and sentiment linking diet and cancer--all of which points to a growing trend toward quality and food safety. Yet these concerns and seeming clamor for a better food system with qualitatively improved practices and products do not automatically add up to carte blanche for biotechnology in the food system.

CONSUMER CONFIDENCE OR CONSUMER FEARS?

Will the new products and farm production aids of agricultural biotechnology enlist consumer confidence, or will consumers be fearful of genetic products in the food and farm system? It's probably too early to answer this question with any clear level of certainty, although some genetically manufactured additives, such as aspartame, are already in the food system.

In at least one area--livestock hormones--we may see some consumer resistance. Given the increasing sensitivity of the general public to the use of hormones and antibiotics in food-producing farm animals, and the December 1985 ban in Europe of steroid hormones in animal husbandry, it is quite possible that consumers will object to, and resist, food products made from animals that have been given genetically engineered hormones.

Four U.S. companies are proceeding with plans to market a genetically engineered bovine growth hormone in the U.S. dairy industry. Meanwhile, a coalition of consumer and dairy farmers in Wisconsin has threatened to conduct an international boycott of all dairy products made from cows treated with such hormones (Smith, 1986).

CONTROL IN THE FOOD SYSTEM

Will biotechnology give consumers more or less control over the foods they eat, and will it give them more or less control over the way food is produced and processed? Again, the simple answer to this question is that biotechnology will probably not give consumers more control over what they eat, and it will certainly not give them more control over the food system as a whole. One reason for this is that consumers will not have any tangible claim on the genes of food production or on the technologies of genetically based food production.

Today, the genes of food production are articles of commerce and are eligible for patenting, as are the technologies--which are remote and inaccessible for the average person to begin with. Rather than giving consumers more control over food production, biotechnology is thus more likely to give the food processing industry greater control over the field-to-table characteristics of food. A July 1986 prospectus for the Calgene Company, which was distributed on Wall Street and throughout the investment community, contains the following statements:

> The unit value of most crops that are grown for the food processing and related industries are

determined primarily by the crops' processing characterisitics, such as texture, flavor, color, protein and carbohydrate content, and shelf life. Food processors have traditionally purchased their plant raw materials, i.e., crops, in commodity markets, where all product is essentially undifferentiated [i.e., as to quality, performance, oil content, etc.]. Plant recombinant DNA technology, however, may provide an opportunity for food processors to gain a competitive advantage by allowing precise genetic modification to develop proprietary crop varieties with enhanced processing characteristics, which can then be patented and grown for their exclusive use (Calgene, Inc., 1986, p. 22).

In America today, roughly 32% of all farm sales are concluded under some form of contract or are vertically integrated by business. The Congressional Office of Technology Assessment, in its March 1986 study of agriculture and technology, made two very interesting points about the extent and expansion of contracting: (1) contracting used to be limited to perishable products, but in recent years has been extended to all commodities, and (2) production contracting appears to be associated with commodities for which breeding and control of genetic factors play an important role in either productivity determination or quality control (U.S. Congress, Office of Technology Assessment, 1986).

In the future, biotechnology may give food processors and shippers a greater power of specificity in contracting with, or buying from, farmers. And for those companies that supply farm inputs, gene-based products--whether in the form of seed, chemicals, or microorganisms--will certainly add a new dimension to their influence over agricultural productivity.

HOW WILL BIOTECHNOLOGY BE APPLIED?

With agricultural biotechnology, research scientists, biotechnology companies, and major food corporations will increasingly determine what is produced in the food system and how it is produced. These practitioners of biotechnology will conduct their work almost exclusively from the confines of the laboratory and the far reaches of the gene. Given this powerful new technology--and the capitalization that will accompany commercially favored applications--some form of regulation and social accountability will be absolutely critical in establishing consumer confidence as well as consumer protection. If it turns out that biotechnologists and food processors are only paying lip service to quality improvements, and are instead using biotechnology predominantly to save money in food processing or to increase their market share in the fruit and vegetable bin by way of biotech-made brands, consumers will have a reason to be wary of this technology and its side effects, just as they have been of other technologies that have come to the food industry in the past.

At this frontier point in the use of genetic technology in the food system, it would be important for a responsible industry to lend its support to government in evaluating the options that are possible for making the food system safer and qualitatively better in all respects, from field to table. Not the least important in this effort would be establishing a workable and reliable monitoring system and data base on nutritional constituents in our raw food resources as well as a good inventory of naturally occurring toxins. This would appear to be the minimum information base needed before all manner of interests go plunging headlong into a free-for-all genetic engineering of the food system.

REFERENCES

Alexander, M. 1985. Ecological consequences: Reducing the uncertainties. Issues Sci. Technol. 1:57-68.

Ames, B.N. 1983. Dietary carcinogens and anticarcinogens. Science 221:1256-1264.

Anderson, D. 1984. Introduction to Phytogen. Phytogen, Pasadena, Calif. 7 pp.

Anonymous. 1982. Kellogg buys stock in seed firm in Denver. Supermarket News, June 7, 1982, p. 8.

Anonymous. 1986. Safeway won't buy apples treated with ripener Alar. Wall Street Journal, July 17, 1986, p. 31.

Associated Press. 1985. Student grows cotton in tube. Journal of Commerce, November 5, 1985, p. 13B.

Brody, J. 1984. Diet to prevent heart attacks aims to cut blood fat levels. New York Times, May 16, 1984, p. A16.

Calgene, Inc. 1986. Prospectus for Public Stock Offering, July 8, 1986. Underwriters: Hambrecht & Quist, Paine Webber, and Piper, Jaffray & Hopwood. Calgene, Inc., Davis, Calif. 59 pp.

Center for Science in the Public Interest. 1986. Americans for Safe Food. Center for Science in the Public Interest, Washington, D.C. 4 pp.

Chavez, C. 1986. Wrath of grapes campaign. Direct mail appeal, May 1986.

Ciba-Geigy Corp. 1986a. Ciba-Geigy seeks approval to conduct small field test of genetically engineered plant. News Release, June 18, 1986. Agricultural Division, Ciba-Geigy Corporation, Greensboro, N.C. 4 pp.

Ciba-Geigy Corp. 1986b. Summary of proposed field test of genetically engineered plants. Special Communication, June 18, 1986. Agricultural Division, Ciba-Geigy Corporation, Greensboro, N.C. 2 pp.

Cox, M. 1982. A french-fry diary: From Idaho furrow to golden arches; for the potato that qualifies, McDonald's has a slicer, sprayer, drier - and ruler. Wall Street Journal, February 8, 1982, p. 1.

Dixon, B. 1986. European steroid ban sparks controversy. Bio/Technol. 4:688.

Doyle, J. 1985a. Altered Harvest: Agriculture, Genetics & the Fate of the World's Food Supply. Viking Penguin, New York. 512 pp.

Doyle, J. 1985b. Biotechnology's harvest of herbicides. GeneWATCH 2:1-2, 14-20.

Doyle, J. 1986. Biotechnology: More herbicides, but at least the crops won't be harmed. J. Pest. Reform 6:26-31.

DNA Plant Technology Corp. 1985. DNAP and Kraft Foods announce agreement to market new vegetable snack products. Press Release, July 19, 1985. Kekst & Co., New York. 2 pp.

DNA Plant Technology Corp. 1986. Prospectus for Public Stock Offering, March 26, 1986. Underwriters: Shearson Lehman Brothers, Inc., and Kidder, Peabody & Co. DNA Plant Technology Corp., Cinnaminson, N.J. 32 pp.

FDA (Food and Drug Administration). 1970. Food Additives: Eligibility of substances for classification as generally recognized as safe in food. Proposed rule. Fed. Regist. 35:18623-18624.

Flynn, J. 1986. Biotechnology: Want some O.J.? It's fresh from the test tube. Bus. Week (2973):160-162.

Gabelman, W.H., J.C. Ayers, F. Haskins, H. Kramer, R.O. Nesheim, W.B. Robinson, N.S. Scrimshaw, and S.H. Wittwer. 1973. Report of the Task Force on Genetic Alterations in Food and Feed Crops. Submitted to the Board on Agriculture and Renewable Resources and the Food and Nutrition Board of the National Academy of Sciences-National Research Council. 16 pp.

Gormley, T.R., G. Downey, and D. O'Beirne. 1986. Technological Change in Agriculture and the Food Industry, and Public Policy in Relation to Food Production, Nutrition and Consumer Safety. Forecasting and Assessment in Science and Technology (FAST), Occasional Papers, No. 107, August 1986. Commission of the European Communities, Brussels. 327 pp.

Hammonds, T. 1985. Public attitudes toward food safety. Agribusiness 1:33-43.

Kellogg Co. 1981. Annual Report, 1981. Kellogg Company, Battle Creek, Mich. 32 pp.

L. William Teweles & Co. 1983. Improved tomatoes: Plant genetic engineering to bear fruit in the 1980s. News Release, December 7, 1983. L. William Teweles & Co., Milwaukee, Wis. 4 pp.

Laster, R. 1986. Remarks of Richard Laster, President and Chief Executive Officer, at DNA Plant Technology Corporation 1986 Annual Stockholders' Meeting, May 7, 1986. DNA Plant Technology Corp., Cinnaminson, N.J. 7 pp.

Lewis, R. 1986. Building a better tomato. High Technol. 6:46-51, 53.

Meier, B. 1986. Heinz to restrict the use in baby foods of crops treated with some chemicals. Wall Street Journal, November 7, 1986, p. 8.

Monsanto Co. 1984. Genetic Engineering: A Natural Science. Monsanto Company, St. Louis. 21 pp.

Morris, B. 1982. Campbell Soup is looking for "super" tomato. Wall Street Journal, April 2, 1982, p. 25.

NRC (National Research Council). 1982. Diet, Nutrition, and Cancer. Report of the Committee on Diet, Nutrition, and Cancer, Assembly of Life Sciences. National Academy Press, Washington, D.C. 496 pp.

Rockefeller Foundation. 1985. The President's Review and Annual Report. Rockefeller Foundation, New York. 145 pp.

Russell, C. 1984. Cancer society starts crusade on U.S. diet. Washington Post, February 11, 1984, p. A1.

Salquist, R.H. 1986. The Future of Biotechnology in Agriculture. Presented at a press briefing sponsored by the Industrial Biotechnology Association (IBA), October 24, 1986, at the IBA Annual Meeting, Westin St. Francis Hotel, San Francisco, California. Industrial Biotechnology Association, Rockville, Md. 9 pp.

Schmeck, H.M., Jr. 1986. Plants "vaccinated" against virus. New York Times, May 6, 1986, p. C1.

Schneiderman, H.A. 1985. Altering the harvest: Biotech's cornucopia. Science '85 6:52, 54.

Shields, M.J. 1985. "Designer" veg on cutting edge. Will "designer" vegetables find the market fertile? Adweek 26(40)National Marketing Edition:1,4.

Smith, K. 1986. Boycott: BGH milk. Agri-View, October 2, 1986, p. B-1.

Spiher, A.T., Jr. 1975. The growing of GRAS (generally recognized as safe). HortScience 10:241-242.

U.S. Congress, Office of Technology Assessment. 1986. Technology, Public Policy, and the Changing Structure of American Agriculture. U.S. Government Printing Office, Washington, D.C. 380 pp.

USDA (U.S. Department of Agriculture). 1970. Notice to Growers of the Withdrawal of the Name of Potato Variety Lenape. Crops Research Division, Agricultural Research Service, U.S. Department of Agriculture, Beltsville, Md. and The Agricultural Experiment Station of Pennsylvania, University Park, Pa. 2 pp.

U.S. Supreme Court. 1980. Syllabus: Diamond, Commissioner of Patents and Trademarks, v. Chakrabarty, No. 79-136. Argued March 17, 1980; decided June 16, 1980. 14 pp.

Zitnak, A., and G.R. Johnston. 1970. Glycoalkaloid content of B5141-6 potatoes. Am. Potato J. 47:256-260.

BIOTECHNOLOGY: ITS POTENTIAL IMPACT ON INTERRELATIONSHIPS AMONG AGRICULTURE, INDUSTRY, AND SOCIETY

Lawrence Busch and William B. Lacy

The last several years have witnessed the beginning of a major change in world agriculture. For the first time in history, patents or patentlike protection have been accorded to plants and even microorganisms. The large agrochemical and pharmaceutical firms have bought many of the world's largest seed companies and have begun to integrate them into their larger plans. Computer technologies and robots have begun to enter into the agricultural sector, changing significantly the ways in which agriculture is managed. Finally, the new biotechnologies have opened new vistas in agriculture, making possible for the first time the engineering of improved plants and animals and promising to make the food processing industries more efficient than ever before. Together, these as yet unrealized technical changes are likely to dwarf the so-called Green Revolution of the 1970s.

In the United States, farmers and the general public tend to view the new biotechnologies favorably. A recent article in American Vegetable Grower is indicative: "The promises of the new developments for agriculture have been widely publicized. For example, the potential and economic impact of new varieties of crops requiring little or no input of costly fertilizer is obvious. Similarly, the development of varieties with better resistance to disease and insects would benefit the production of many crops" (Boyer, 1984, p. 51). Unfortunately, our review of the literature and interviews with scientists suggest that the author's enthusiasm is at best likely to be short-lived.

In this paper we review these changes with specific emphasis on biotechnology. Of concern here is how the new biotechnologies, and the social and scientific changes that they engender, are likely to be used by powerful interests to change what we eat. In the past, agriculture has been different from manufacturing, in part because of its need for land and its dependence upon seasonal changes. Lenin noted that "agriculture possesses certain features which cannot possibly be removed (if we leave aside the extremely problematical possibility of producing albumen and foods by artificial processes)" (Lenin, 1938, p. 85). Yet, it appears that just such a possibility is upon the horizon. Is it possible that biotechnology will create a world of superabundant food? Is hunger to be finally eliminated as a part of the human condition? Or are there other forces that will shape the biotechnology revolution to other ends?

SAVING THE METAPHOR

Plant biology has, until recently, rarely descended below the level of the plant organ or part. This was in part a result of lower levels of funding, but was also due to the greater difficulties of working with plant cells and the strong applied character of the plant sciences. Conventional plant breeding--what we may refer to as the old biotechnologies--has proceeded with some help from Mendelian genetics, but with a heavy and necessary dose of empiricism.[1] It has five basic steps: (1) the discovery or creation of genetically stable variation for the desired traits; (2) selection of individuals best expressing those traits; (3) incorporation of the traits into a desirable agronomic background; (4) testing over a wide range of habitats and several seasons; and (5) the release of the new variety.

In the last decade, however, it has become possible to apply techniques developed for molecular biology to plant improvement. These techniques can be divided into two

---

[1] For a more detailed review of both conventional and new techniques of plant improvement, see Hansen et al. (1986).

broad classes: culturing and genetic transfer. Culturing involves the regeneration of plants from protoplasts (plant cells with the cell wall removed), single cells, or plant parts. These culturing techniques have three advantages over conventional approaches: (1) One can grow an enormous number of different cells, each a potential plant, in a small area. (2) The process of sexual reproduction can be more easily bypassed, thereby allowing access to genetic material that is inaccessible through the propagation of gametes and eliminating the delay necessary for multigenerational change. (3) The mass screening of plant material can be accomplished in a very short time; for example, a harmful substance can be added to the culture so that only resistant cells grow. There is a problem with these techniques, however: What is expressed at the level of the single cell may not be expressed at the level of the whole plant. In addition, only those traits for which a cellular analog exists can be selected with these techniques; important traits such as root strength, resistance to lodging, and other whole plant characteristics are not amenable to these selection procedures.

In contrast to culture techniques, genetic transfer techniques operate at the single cell, subcellular, or molecular levels. Transfer may be either general or specific. General transfer involves fusion of protoplasts or transfer of specific organelles. Specific transfer depends upon the recombinant DNA technologies. A specific piece of genetic information is transferred and expressed in the host. For example, the genetic material conferring herbicide tolerance has been transferred and expressed in a crop plant. This permits spraying for weeds without damaging the crop. Widespread use of this technique offers precision and control that is simply unavailable through culture techniques. In principle, breeders could transfer just the genes that they desire. The major limitation on recombinant techniques is the lack of information on the location and function of the genes of higher plants. Moreover, the most agronomically interesting techniques are multigenic; it is not yet clear just how these traits are expressed.

Most of these difficulties went unrecognized by early proponents of plant molecular biology. They often perceived plants as the same as microorganisms. As Chaleff explains: "With recognition of the similarities between cultured plant cells and microorganisms came the expectation that all the extraordinary feats of genetic experimentation accomplished with microbes would soon be realized with plants. But because of the many ways in which cultured plant cells are unlike microbes, these expectations thus far have not been well-fulfilled" (Chaleff, 1983, p. 679; see also Schaeffer and Sharpe, 1983). In short, early proponents of plant molecular biology took their own metaphor literally. That is, they believed that the metaphorical equivalence (plant = microorganism) was actually the case.

Despite this confusion, plant molecular biology has been a growth industry. Large sums of money have been invested by various public authorities, by large petrochemical and pharmaceutical firms, and, especially in the United States where laws are particularly favorable, by many small venture capital firms. Moreover, since the venture capital firms could survive only by attracting large sums of capital, they soon became the greatest defenders of the metaphor. The hype found in their prospectuses succeeded not only in attracting capital, but also convinced many in the public sector of the validity of the metaphor.

Although no major breakthroughs have occurred, great progress has been made in developing plants tolerant to glyphosate (a major herbicide). This is of enormous commercial potential to the companies involved. On the other hand, many of the venture capital firms have gone bankrupt, while others have been bought by the petrochemical or pharmaceutical giants. Only a handful have been able to generate some salable product and thereby also generate additional capital.

Our story does not end here, however. Although whole plants are much more complicated than microorganisms and pose many problems for molecular biologists, the metaphor might yet be saved if the focus of research were to change. Instead of centering on the improvement of plants in the field, plant cells could be treated as if they were microorganisms. The techniques of growth and fermentation of bacteria, already well known to certain segments of the food processing industry (especially cheese and bread making and alcohol production), combined with the newer techniques of cell culture could be used to transform the production of certain agricultural commodities into industrial processes.

In principle, any commodity that is consumed in an undifferentiated or highly processed form could be produced in this manner. Similarly, though with greater difficulty, tissue culture techniques could be used to produce edible plant parts in vitro. In short, agricultural production in the field would be supplanted by cell and tissue culture factories. Lenin's (1938) dream of the complete elimination of agriculture and its replacement with continuous process factory production would at last be fulfilled!

Of course, the transformation we have just described is not likely to take place within the next year or even the next decade. Indeed, it is difficult to say which research trajectories will be developed and which will be abandoned. Undoubtedly, the ways in which markets for food products and processes are organized, the regulatory requirements imposed on the industry, and the scope of patent laws will play a major role in determining just how and how much the food system is reorganized. However, the scientific foundations for change are now being laid. Consider the following:

• Markets for certain tropical commodities have already been restructured. Sugar, once an extremely important tropical commodity, has already been hard hit by the development of corn sweeteners and sugar substitutes such as aspartame (Nutrasweet). It is unlikely that the sugar market will recover from its current state of overproduction and depression. It has been estimated that the livelihood of 8 million to 10 million people in the Third World has been threatened as a result (van den Doel and Junne, 1986).

A similar change has occurred with respect to the production of cooking oils; corn oil has become a major ingredient in prepared foods in developed countries. In addition, food processing techniques have been modified to make it possible to substitute oils in processing if desirable because of relative market prices. Thus, it is now common in the United States to see notes on bread packages indicating that one or more different oils may be used in the manufacturing process. In economic terms, the cross-elasticities of cooking oils have increased.

One of the first crops to be affected by tissue culture research was oil palm. The multinational Unilever Corporation, owner of large oil palm plantations in Malaysia and elsewhere, realized in the 1960s the potential for tissue culture of oil palm (James, 1984).[2] Unlike many other tropical commodities, there had been little work to improve oil palm; at the same time, there was great genetic variation among trees. The actual research was conducted in Britain in greenhouses. Palm oil production was increased 30% by using tissue culture techniques to clone high-yielding trees. As of 1984, 12,000 improved trees had been planted. In addition, "more uniform, shorter trees facilitate mechanization of harvesting, reducing labor costs" (van den Doel and Junne, 1986, p. 88). Given that approximately 30 million trees must be replanted annually, there is likely to be a steady market for the clones.

Moreover, since palm oil producers now compete with producers of other oils such as coconut, soy, olive, and cottonseed oils, the increased production of palm oil has had the effect of reducing demand for these other oils. American soybean producers are painfully aware of this. Similarly, in the Philippines where fully 25% of the population is at least partially dependent upon coconut production for their livelihood, oil production and export has dropped precipitously in recent years (Bijman et al., 1986). Although estimates of labor displacment in that country are virtually unobtainable, it is clear that it has been extensive. Furthermore, as more countries adopt the higher yielding palm clones, it is likely that the price will be depressed to near or below production costs.

Still another area of important scientific advance is the production of what food technologists call fabricated

---

[2] In contrast, little work has been done to improve coconut oil production, in part because the 60 million persons worldwide involved in this industry are largely smallholders (Bijman et al., 1986).

foods. Such foods (often developed from soybeans) "differ from conventional foods in that their basic components--proteins, fats, and carbohydrates--may be derived from many sources and combined, along with the necessary micro-nutrients, flavors, and colors, to form an attractive product" (Stanley, 1986, p. 65). The consumer may not even be able to identify the origin of these foods.

• Work is currently under way to produce the flavor components of expensive fragrances, spices, and flavoring agents through tissue culture (see Table 1). As Collin and Watts (1983) stated:

> Many of the compounds are obtained from plants that are not grown under large-scale or controlled cultivation. This instability, combined with climatic, harvesting, transport difficulties, and possible political problems in the country of origin, often leads to considerable fluctuations in the price of the compound. With each of these compounds there is interest in a more stable and easily controlled source (Collin and Watts, 1983, pp. 731-732).

As one proponent put it, "The research and development effort required is well worth the effort to achieve the *in vitro* production of not only specialty biochemicals, but potentially, food, spices, and industrial commodities" (Staba, 1985, p. 203). Wheat (1986) reported that a number of major corporations and biotechnology companies are currently using this approach to create products such as fruit-based flavors, mint oil, quinine, and saffron. In addition, work is apparently in progress to produce coffee, cocoa, rubber, and tea *in vitro* (Clairmonte and Cavanagh, 1986; Heinstein, 1985; Staba, 1985; Tsai and Kinsella, 1981). Citrus pulp vesicles have also been produced *in vitro*, thereby presenting the possibility that fresh orange juice could be produced daily (Rogoff and Rawlins, 1987). These flavor components would be identical biochemically to the compounds naturally found in these products; hence, they would not be artificial in the sense now understood but would be true equivalents.

• Also important is the factory production of pharmaceuticals and industrial chemicals using tissue culture techniques (e.g., Anderson et al., 1985; Breuling et al., 1985; Dixon, 1984; Misawa, 1985; Rosevear and Lambe, 1985;

TABLE 1 Markets for Selected Plant Products[a]

Plant or Compound	Use/Product	Wholesale Price, U.S.$/kg	Estimated World Demand, millions of U.S. $
Vinblastine	Medication for leukemia	5,000	18-20[b]
Jasmine	Flavor; fragrance	5,000	0.5[b]
Catharanthus	Vincristine	5,000	18-20[b]
Lithospermum	Shikonin	4,500	c
Digitalis	Medication for heart disorders	3,000	20-55[b]
Rose Otto	Rose oil	2,800	12
Ajmalicine	Medication for circulatory problems	1,500	5.25
Papaver	Codeine	650	50[b]
Pyrethrins	Insecticide	300	20[b]
Buchu	Buchu oil	220	153
Cinnamon	Flavor	195	3.2
Quinine	Medication for malaria; flavor	100	5-10[b]
Ginger	Flavor	100	33
Spearmint	Flavor; fragrance	30	85-90
Sapota	Chicle	c	c
Cinchona	Quinine	c	20-55[b]
Coffee	Beverage	12	2,210
Cocoa	Beverage; flavor	4	891
Tea	Beverage	2	2,917
Rubber	Tires and other products	1	3,565

[a]From Collin and Watts, 1983; Curtin, 1983; FAO, 1985; Kenney et al., 1984.
[b]U.S. market only.
[c]Not known.

Yamada, 1984; Yamada and Fujita, 1983). Many of these are secondary metabolites of plants, which are extremely expensive--often selling for more than $2,000 per kilogram. They are used in various processes to produce dyes, astringents, pharmaceuticals (more than 25% of the prescriptions filled in the United States are for drugs derived from plants [Balandrin et al., 1985]), and other rare but essential industrial or consumer goods. Balandrin and colleagues link in vitro production with political instabilities:

> As the natural habitats for wild plants disappear and environmental and political instabilities make it difficult to acquire plant derived chemicals, it may become necessary to develop alternative sources for important plant products. There has been considerable interest in plant cell culture as a potential alternative to traditional agriculture for the industrial production of secondary plant metabolites. This has given rise to considerable research in Japan, West Germany, and Canada (Balandrin et al., 1985, p. 1158).

Misawa (1985) makes a similar case, while noting the similarity between tissue culture and microbial fermentations. He also observed that such in vitro techniques permit production "in any place or season" (Misawa, 1985, p. 60). According to him, four types of products are of interest: alkaloids and steroids for pharmaceuticals, terpenoids as antitumor compounds, and quinones as drugs against heart disease. Systems as large as 20,000 liters--large by scientific, but still small by industrial, standards--have been built (Fowler, 1984). Production costs are still too high for the use of these techniques with foodstuffs.

This interest has given rise to tissue culture-based manufacturing plants in both West Germany and Japan. Balandrin et al. (1985) estimated that such processes are economical when cultures produce one gram of the desired compound per liter of culture and the selling price is between $500 and $1,000 per kilogram. Among the advantages for culture techniques are standard growth conditions, less complex organization than the entire plant, and ease of purifying the desired product (Anderson et al., 1985). Moreover, the heterogeneity of cultured plant cells makes possible the selection and multiplication of those with the highest yield. Culture techniques also offer the potential to create entirely new products either through the collection of newly discovered, naturally occurring compounds or through the manipulation of cells to make them produce entirely new compounds.

Consider the claim made by Yamada and Fujita (1983) for a dye/astringent currently being produced in Japan:

> Compared with shikon requiring 2-3 years for harvest of the plant, cultured cells permit harvesting within about three weeks, thereby greatly shortening the production period. The content of the shikonin[3] derivatives in the cultured cells was about 14%, which was extremely high compared with 1-2% in the normal field grown shikon (Yamada and Fujita, 1983, p. 726).

Shikonin is now selling for more than $4,000 per kilogram. One ironic note is that the in vitro production may actually drive the price down too rapidly, given the fact that the market is small and easy to saturate (Curtin, 1983).

There are persistent, but unconfirmed rumors within the genetic engineering community that at least one U.S. company has mounted a program to produce tomato pulp in vitro. This technique would be used to produce an array of canned tomato products, including sauce, paste, catsup, and puree. Similarly, there are rumors that a French company has already produced apple sauce in vitro and is now attempting to scale up the process for industrial production.

• As noted above, the final stage of biotechnology involves the replacement of agricultural processes with industrial processes. Here, too, much initial work has been accomplished. Cotton fibers have been grown directly from cotton cells. Unlike those produced in the field, test tube fibers can grow from both ends. Although it is

---

[3] Shikonin is the chemical product derived from the shikon plant.

unlikely that field production will be replaced in the near future, the potential is there (Anonymous, 1986).[4]

Similarly, the Japan Salt and Tobacco Public Corporation and Plant Science Limited of the United Kingdom are both investigating the in vitro production of tobacco biomass for cigarettes (Curtin, 1983). Thus far, the processes have proved too expensive for commercial use.

• Perhaps the most far-reaching proposal to replace agriculture is that found in a paper by Rogoff and Rawlins (1987). They propose a system in which most fields are planted with perennial crops grown for biomass. These crops would be harvested as needed and turned into sugar by using enzymes at the point of harvest. The sugar solution is then piped to production plants in metropolitan areas. Finally, food is produced through massively scaled-up tissue cultures by using sugar solution as a medium and nutrient source for the plant material. As they put it, "In this strategy, edible products are synthesized from separately manufactured food components, plant (and animal) parts, or biological derivatives manufactured in vitro" (Rogoff and Rawlins, 1987, p. 801). Under this system, processing would be a year-round activity in which only that actually needed would be produced on a given day. Canning and freezing would be largely eliminated as would most spoilage, since food would be produced and consumed in the same general vicinity. In fact, the same production facility could be shifted from the production of one commodity to another in response to changing demand.

Rogoff and Rawlins argue that such a system would have other added benefits in terms of reduced need of monocropping, lowered soil erosion, less use of agrichemicals, reduced energy inputs, and minimal transportation costs. They go on to note that the work necessary to realize this

---

[4]Wittwer (1985) has noted that pyrethrin--the natural insecticidal component of some plants--can, as a result of plant improvement using the methods of tissue culture, now be grown more cheaply in the field than by synthesis in the laboratory. This should give us cause to withhold any simplistic generalizations about the role of tissue culture in replacing crops in the field.

scenario is already under way but that it is currently uncoordinated, and they suggest a number of ways to bring about a more coordinated strategy.

The major stumbling block to such a transformation of the world food system is the production costs involved (Zenk, 1978). For example, the sugar solution would have to be produced at a considerably lower cost than now possible before this technology could be reasonably adopted on a large scale. Yet, Rogoff and Rawlins (1987) point out that transport costs would decline so much that production costs could double without significantly altering the final price. Moreover, it is unlikely that the switch to such a system would take place all at once. It takes little imagination to realize that costs are likely to become competitive with conventional production methods when the product is a luxury good available only in limited quantities or when it is heavy and produced far from its point of consumption. In both instances, cell and tissue culture techniques offer significant advantages. On the other hand, there are forces that will inhibit the rapid development of in vitro production. In particular, it appears likely that large, multinational enterprises will resist the rapid demise of the lucrative markets that they now dominate. In these instances, they will intervene by defensive patenting, by purchasing potential biotechnological competitors, or by supporting government regulation of the competition. Indeed, Byé and Mounier (1984) suggested that this is precisely why the otherwise desirable in vitro production of proteins (largely for animal production) has not become feasible.

Since Third World nations rarely own large shares of multinational companies, products that they produce and that cannot be produced in the field in more developed countries are likely to become targets of biotechnological research. In addition, Third World countries are much more vulnerable to these production shifts than are those of the First or Second Worlds.

FROM INSTRUMENTS TO PRODUCTION TECHNIQUES

Before the probable impacts of such changes can be examined, it is important to clarify the central role played by science and technology. Traditionally, sociologists, philosophers, and historians of science have viewed science as a quest for new ideas. They have paid scant attention to the central importance of instruments in modern science (cf. Busch, 1984; Ihde, 1979; Laudan, 1984). Yet, it is obvious to even the most casual observer of a scientific laboratory that instruments are central to the process of doing science. Moreover, like the rest of us, scientists always work under fiscal constraints. This is true of even the most well-supported scientists. As a result, they are always seeking new ways to cut the costs of their work, so that they might accomplish more with the same amount of money. In this respect, then, scientists are much like capitalists; although they seek credit (profits?) in the form of publications and citations, rather than money, they are inexorably driven to reduce the cost of scientific production as surely as the capitalist is driven to reduce the production cost of goods and services.

When this process is applied to plant molecular biology, we can immediately see its importance. Plant molecular biologists are interested in understanding the ways in which plant genetic material is structured. Even if they have little or no interest in the commercial opportunities presented by improved seeds, they need to have rapid, efficient methods for moving from individual protoplasts or cells to tissue to whole plants in order to ensure that what is created at the molecular or cellular level is expressed in the whole plant.

The various techniques for plant improvement described above are nested, as illustrated in Figure 1. Recombinant techniques may be used to transfer a specific gene to a plant cell. That cell must then be cultured into a tissue. The tissue in turn must be differentiated into a plantlet (excluding for the moment the possibility of in vitro production). The plant must be tried in the field to learn if the trait incorporated at the molecular level is expressed in a field setting. Finally, the new cultivar must be multiplied and released. If any of the steps in this process are impossible or difficult, they will be a bottleneck to the whole process.

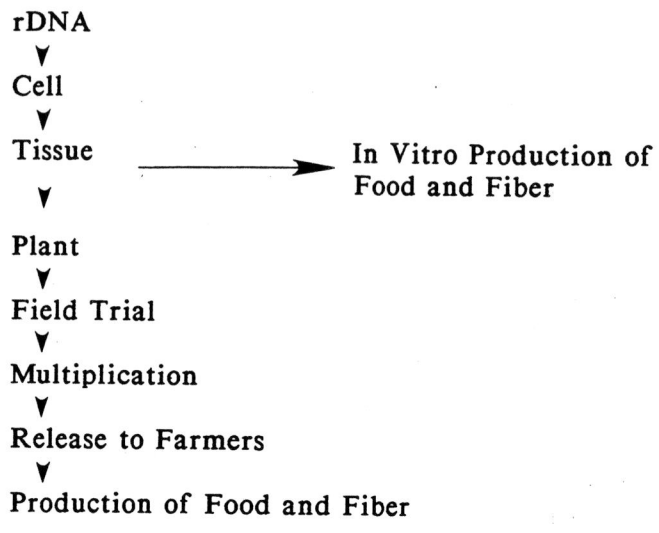

FIGURE 1 Steps involved in plant improvement and production using conventional techniques and the new biotechnologies.

This creates an enormous incentive to improve culturing processes. A recent article appropriately entitled "Assembly Line Plants Take Root" provides an example:

> The biggest thing keeping costs up--and therefore holding tissue culture propagation back-- is the amount of labor needed to run a tissue-culture lab. . . . Automation is one solution to the problem of high labor costs. ARS [Agricultural Research Service] scientists in California have found a way to automate their tissue-culture work and at the same time achieve at least two to four times the growth rate of traditional tissueculture systems. Plant geneticist Brent Tisserat and chemist Carl E. Vandercook use a computer to control the flow of liquid nutrients to plantlets (Comis and Wood, 1986, p. 10)

In addition, Daly (1985) has noted that automated DNA synthesizers are already in use in both academia and industry. Elsewhere, similar efforts are under way to make more efficient the plant improvement process. In short, the very development of scientific techniques and equipment for use in the improvement of conventional agriculture makes possible the elimination of agriculture as we know it. The metaphor, plant = microorganisms, can be saved by restructuring the process of plant improvement so that the culturing process produces the final product in terms of food or fiber; the field as a location for food and fiber production would then cease to exist. As one scientist, Don Dougall, put it, "We have to stop thinking of these things as plant cells, and start thinking of them as new microorganisms, with all the potential that implies" (interview quoted in Curtin, 1983, p. 657).

CONSEQUENCES

Market Restructuring

Even if just a few of the research programs described above were to be brought to fruition, major restructurings would occur. In the United States and Western Europe, the effects would be important but relatively minor, since the farm population is already quite small and other employment opportunities exist for at least some of those displaced. However, it is well known that many Third World countries are dependent upon one or two agricultural commodities for their continued economic stability. Let us examine the impact of biotechnological replacements for one major tropical commodity--rubber.

Chamala (1985) reported that 75% of the world's rubber comes from Malaysia and Indonesia. In Malaysia, 500,000 smallholders are directly engaged in rubber production and 3 million persons--approximately one-quarter of the total population--are directly or indirectly dependent upon it. In Indonesia, the estimated number of dependent people is 8 million. Smallholder rubber producers are among the poorest inhabitants of both countries. Worldwide, an estimated 22 million people depend on the rubber industry. If in vitro production of rubber or the use of tissue culture to improve guayule (a rubber source that grows in temperate climates) (Fisher, 1986; Radin et al., 1982) were to become a reality, 90 to 95% of these people would find themselves without a cash crop (assuming the other 5 to 10% would continue to grow rubber for domestic and specialized uses). Given that the unemployment rates in Malaysia and Indonesia are already high, it would be unlikely that more than 20% of those displaced (about 4 million people) would find alternative employment. Some estimated 16 million people, with few or no marketable skills would find themselves without work or reduced to bare subsistence farming. This is a conservative estimate. Similar effects can be expected for other tropical commodities.

The market restructurings likely to be caused by significant in vitro production or the collapse of existing markets would be enormous. Not only is it likely that a significant number of farmers and farmworkers would find themselves with no products to sell, even many of the traditional agribusiness giants might discover that their huge investments were no longer profitable.

Moreover, although markets may be protected from product competition, little or no protection is provided by new technology (Vergopoulos, 1985). As in vitro and other substitutes are developed, they are likely to lead to the rapid demise of existing commodity markets, as processors restructure their production toward the new input. Without some international system of regulation and compensation, the effects on particular countries are likely to be just short of catastrophic.

The degree of impact can be estimated by looking at past instances of market collapse. For example, Mexico used to grow large quantities of barbasco, a plant from which steroids can be produced. Today, barbasco is no longer grown; the large, pharmaceutical companies have developed a method of producing it chemically, without need for the plant (Dembo et al., 1985). In the more distant past is the demise of the indigo industry in India. In 1897, 574,000 hectares of indigo were grown. By 1920, with the successful development of a chemically produced indigo, field production had all but ceased. Although the planters attempted to develop a research fund in order to compete with chemically produced indigo, they ultimately failed to do so (Martin-Leake, 1975). The result, for that region of India, was widespread depression and unemployment (Kenney et al., 1984).

Every time farmers and farmworkers are displaced, they migrate to urban areas in search of work. Men often leave their wives and families behind to engage in subsistance farming. If the scenario developed herein takes place, the same pattern could occur on a massive scale. The impact could be particularly hard on women and children, for they are likely to bear the full brunt of market restructuring.

Market restructuring affects not only the producers of the primary product but also those engaged in the transport, processing, and even retailing of the final product. Thus, cumulative effects are likely to be much greater than would be the case if changes were somehow limited to farm production. Among the possible effects are geographic shifts in the location of the production process, the demise or growth of secondary industries, secondary effects that result from the inability of the former producing countries to afford importation of various manufactured goods, and the decline of certain consumer goods industries in the Third World as demand declines.

Finally, it requires no crystal ball to realize that a very significant effect of the new biotechnologies in agriculture may be a shift in the geographic location of agricultural production from the Third to the First World. This in turn could create an increase in the already high Third World debt and a concomitant deficit in the balance of payments in Third World countries. Its effects are likely to be felt even more strongly in the West. Major bank failures in the West are a possibility and could be triggered by market restructuring. Moreover, we can safely assume that the major banks will not be allowed to fail, but will be bailed out by the national banks of the Western powers. This in turn will tend to raise taxes and national debts in the West.

Third World Science

In recent years, certain Third World nations--for example, India and Brazil--have succeeded in establishing successful agricultural scientific communities. However, the scientists in those communities have only recently begun to develop products that can make a substantial difference in their respective agricultural economies. They have been aided in this endeavor by the International Agricultural Research Centers and bilateral aid agreements that have provided training and support. Nevertheless, Third World science has often tended to be derivative in character (Chatelin, 1986). It has not entered uncharted areas but has been content to take care of the details in the well-charted parts of nature (Goonatilake, 1982). It has avoided the so-called basic sciences on the grounds--usually supported by First World donors--that all basic science is an expensive luxury. As Goldstein stated, "Original scientists in underdeveloped countries work in a social vacuum, and their activities are too often regarded as useless" (Goldstein, 1988, p. 322). According to Chatelin and Arvanitis (1984), the Third World has been characterized by "scientific domination."

As a result, even in Third World nations with scientific communities, few scientists are capable of pursuing the paths opened by the new biotechnologies. Only a few Third World nations have the critical mass of scientists necessary to engage in genetic engineering; a somewhat larger number may be able to use tissue culture techniques for selected crops. None will be able to mount the broad research campaign needed even to stay abreast of the First World countries. While the International Center for Biotechnology, supported by United Nations Industrial Development Organization, might help in some small ways, it is not likely to be able to assume the role played by the International Agricultural Research Centers in supporting the research that led to the Green Revolution.

The rapid worldwide growth of technical personnel in this area is also worthy of note. For example, in 1931 only two persons were working with plant tissue culture; now there are more than 10,000 (Gautheret, 1983), nearly all of whom are located in the developed world. Salaries for such people are high, and training programs are still relatively few. Only a handful of developing countries will be able to afford to create a critical mass of scientists in this area.

Access to final products as well as to the processes used to produce them is another concern. The new technologies generated by the Green Revolution were created in the public sector and access to them was relatively unproblematic. In contrast, much of the biorevolution is likely to be shrouded in secrecy or patents. This is particularly true in the United States. As Curtin puts it: "Companies tend to be more close-mouthed about their activities in plant tissue culture than they are about culturing mammalian cells, especially in the United States. Elsewhere--in Western Europe and, most notably in Japan--their interest is more substantial and more obvious" (Curtin, 1983, p. 649). Even Europeans are concerned about the potential consequences of being cut off from U.S. biotechnology research (European Economic Community, 1986). This secrecy means that the biorevolution is likely to appear with shocking immediacy as once-stable markets collapse and market shares are suddenly rearranged.

Moreover, the Green Revolution was spatially limited by the very nature of the crops involved (Buttel and Barker, 1985). The biorevolution will not be spatially limited, even if factory production of food remains an elusive goal for some. In principle, recombinant and tissue culture techniques can be used and, in practice, applied to an increasing extent to all crops. Moreover, these same techniques can be used to extend the growing regions of crops, to increase crop substitutability, and to develop crops that have "functional properties" (Moshy, 1986) that make them particularly amenable to certain processing, packaging, nutritional, or aesthetic uses. Bijman and colleagues argued, "Those farms and regions which already have a technological advantage will be the first to benefit from the application of biotechnology. The gap between large and small, rich and poor, and between North and South will thus be widened" (Bijman et al., 1986, p. 22).

In addition, even if the Third World nations are able to develop a cadre of trained scientists, they must also overcome the barriers currently restricting access to the instruments, supplies, and materials needed to do biotechnological research. Without this, at best they can copy some of the less imaginative efforts of the West. As Baltimore (1982) explained:

> However, the training and the ability to self-define problems were coupled to an infrastructure of supply companies that provided specialized equipment such as centrifuges; enzymes, which are the heart of the technology; fine chemicals; laboratory gadgetry, some of which is crucial to research; specialized chromatography media; and so on. The infrastructure is possibly the most crucial part of the system (Baltimore, 1982, p. 33).

Moreover, no research group can manufacture all the chemicals it needs--or even most of them--by itself. It must depend upon commercial suppliers located far from the site of the research. Many of these materials--especially the enzymes--are fragile, must be shipped under special conditions, and must be delivered within several days. For example, one large U.S. supplier of enzymes, the Sigma-Alrich Corporation, was able to sell $215 million in chemicals in 1985, almost entirely by mail. The company reported that 97% of their orders are shipped within 24 hours of receipt (Simon, 1986). Most Third World countries will have great difficulty in linking their scientists to such a supply system.

Let us assume, however, that the Third World is successful in mounting the expertise necessary to develop its own biotechnology research competence. This might be of some small help in offsetting the collapse of various commodity markets. In some cases, patents developed in the Third World might even prevent developed countries from capturing certain markets. Tissue culture might be used to reduce production costs of field-grown crops, thereby making competition from *in vitro* production that much more difficult. However, although this might slow down the changes, it would in no way prevent the loss of millions of jobs in agricultural production. In short, the development of Third World science is no solution to the destabilizing effects of biotechnology.

Political Stability

The use of the new biotechnologies in the production of food is very likely to increase political instability. In the Third World, it could dash the hopes of many who yearn for a better life. Although some persons would undoubtedly revert to food crop production on land used for industrial crops, popular upheavals are likely to occur as displaced populations demand that their fragile states provide food and shelter. Political instability could also occur in the First World, as a result of bank failures, higher taxes, and the elimination of certain processing and transport industries. In both the First and Third Worlds, it is likely that the changes forecast here would create additional social stratification, a greater gap between the rich and the poor, and greater possibilities for class conflict.

Nutrition and Food Safety

It also appears unlikely that the new biotechnologies will be without effects on both nutrition and food safety. For those who are displaced, the spectre of hunger may loom ever larger. Somehow, there is a continuing failure among scientists to realize that the production of more food does not necessarily lead to the elimination of hunger. Hunger can only be eliminated when everyone has the wherewithal to obtain the means of subsistence, whether through access to land on which to grow food or to money to purchase it.

For those in the Third World who do have enough to eat and for those in the First World who become consumers of food modified by the new biotechnologies or produced in vitro, the problem is somewhat different. We now know that human nutrition depends upon the daily ingestion of certain nutrients, although there is some disagreement about the precise quantities needed. In general, we can say with some confidence that we know the quantities of the micronutrients that we need to consume but that we have somewhat greater difficulty determining the levels of macronutrients. Considerable disagreement exists concerning the recommended daily allowances for fats and carbohydrates. This is in part due to the difficulty of conducting tests on human beings as well as to the complex interdependence among nutrients. We know even less about the interactions among foods or between foods and adulterants.

This all adds up to a very large question mark. Every time that we eat fresh foods, we ingest unknown quantities of unknown soil bacteria. Do these play a role in our diet? Every plant product that we eat is itself the result of the peculiar circumstances that happen to exist in a particular field. This in turn affects the chemical composition, flavor, and texture of the things we eat. Normally, we eat a variety of foods that derive their nutrient content as a result of these different field conditions. Moreover, we normally ingest small quantities of substances that are toxic in large quantities. We know little about the role these compounds play in nutrition. As Ronk suggested, even "increasing the amount of an essential nutrient in a particular food may be beneficial in theory, but not in practice if it predisposes the food to growth of either pathogenic or spoilage bacteria, or if it interferes with another nutrient" (Ronk, 1986, pp. 30-31).

Food products that incorporate genetic material from exotic sources, or entirely eliminate toxic substances, especially food products produced in vitro, would reduce the diverse range of ingredients in our food supply and perhaps eliminate many of them. Yet, it is highly questionable whether we have the necessary knowledge to construct artificially a large portion of our food supply. Would such a food supply be adequate, not only in the short run but also in the very long run? What effects might it have after several generations?

Unfortunately, the present state of science fails in its attempts to answer these questions. Indeed, it appears that they are very difficult if not impossible to raise. Consider the following:

● There is a sharp break between the food and nutrition area and that of agricultural production (see Randolph and Sachs, 1981). This gap extends from the U.S. National Academy of Sciences, where food and nutrition are in one board and agriculture in another, to the structure of most universities, where colleges of agriculture are often separate from schools of nutrition.

● Both the agricultural and nutrition sciences tend toward reductionism. That is, they tend to assume that the world can be subdivided into a series of discrete problems that can be resolved serially. Without a doubt, for some problems this type of approach can and does work quite well. However, for other problems, such as those raised here, reductionist strategies fail to grasp the problem.

● Even now the testing of new food products and food additives is a complex and arduous task with which few governments are able to cope adequately. The production of food and drug products with the aid of the new biotechnologies will undoubtedly put added stress on a system that is at best a weak one. Will these products be considered the same as food produced in the traditional ways and thus escape government testing? Or will they be considered new and require elaborate test methods? (They are likely to be considered new for the purpose of patenting). If they are to be tested, how stringent should these tests be? Indeed, can tests be devised for potential problems that are chronic rather than acute?

• In both nutrition and food science, emphasis is not placed on the development of informed policies. In nutrition, the focus is the clinical diagnosis of problems; in food science, it is the development of new food products and processes. Members of both sciences often studiously avoid food policy questions on the grounds that they lie outside their domains. Yet, de facto, the very products that they develop create a food policy. And who has the expertise in these areas if not those in the scientific community?

• An additional problem is the need to protect our food from contamination. Even today, for all food produced in the field, there are occasional documented cases of contamination of food products, either by accident, by a misguided or deranged individual, or even for political reasons. However, the production of food or food ingredients in vitro creates much greater security problems. Contamination of large quantities of food--for whatever reason--is easier when there is in vitro production, simply because so much food is produced in so small an area. Moreover, protection of such production facilities would be difficult and would necessitate undemocratic institutional forms. Given that some observers have encouraged in vitro production as a remedy for political turmoil, this problem presents both ironies and contradictions.

CONCLUSIONS

There is a certain irony in that the technological optimism described above is associated with social pessimism. As noted, however, even technological optimism must be examined carefully. Despite impressions to the contrary, this is an extremely difficult task. The only source of information about future directions in biotechnological research is the scientific community itself. That community is strongly biased in the direction of technological optimism. Some years ago, for example, scientists were infatuated with the prospect of modifying plant materials through irradiation, and a little later we were told that the sea would provide the abundant food supply needed for future generations. Neither of these predictions have come to pass. Current forecasts for _in vitro_ production pay little attention to the intricate and expensive basic scientific research that must still be conducted in order to modify even the simplest plant characteristics (e.g., studies to unravel the plant nutrition process and the relationship of some plant parts to the development of flavor in the edible parts), the complex developmental research necessary to arrive at production prototypes, the difficulties of scale-up (e.g., Senior, 1986), and the economics of large-scale production (Goldstein, 1983). These are likely to be formidable barriers. However, even though the prognostications provided by scientists may be biased, we can ignore them only at our peril. The possibility exists that a radical restructuring of what we now call agriculture could be triggered by powerful interests using these technologies. We must examine the likely consequences now and ask whether we wish to pursue this path. Yet at the same time, we must remain skeptics.

On the other hand, the new biotechnologies offer us an opportunity to assess new technology before it actually exists. This is particularly desirable in that it permits--at least in principle--the avoidance of deleterious effects of proposed technical change through the reorganization of markets and the creation of governmental and intergovernmental policies to direct that change. Much still needs to be done, however. A more careful review and monitoring of the scientific literature are essential. In addition, more detailed forecasts of the impact of particular technical changes are needed.

Nevertheless, we can make some fairly strong statements about impacts if we accept the optimistic position that some scientists provide to us. First, we can expect a major transformation of agriculture over the next quarter century. Specifically, we can expect the not-so-gradual breakdown of spatial, temporal, and climatic barriers to food and fiber production. This alone will bring with it substantial social upheavals as the location of production changes. In addition, we can expect the elimination of major portions of the farming enterprise if field crops are grown _in vitro_. This in turn will displace farmers and farmworkers on a scale never before possible. Moreover, most of these tens or perhaps hundreds of millions of persons will not be able to find work in other sectors of the world economy. Thus, the demise of agriculture would deprive many of the very means of subsistence. Another aspect of the new biotechnologies is the enormous concentration of economic and therefore political power that it is likely to make possible. Linkages between the chemical, pharmaceutical, seed, and food industries have already been formed. Concentrated production would also bring with it the possibility of deliberate or accidental contamination of the food supply; in a word, it would actually reduce our food security.

We need not believe that the new biotechnologies must inevitably lead us in certain directions and that things could not possibly be otherwise. We have both options and responsibilities. Let us consider some of them.

• Although we have spent millions to develop research capacity in the new biotechnologies, we have not supported research on their broader consequences. Yet it appears not unreasonable to ask that scientists assess the potential impact of their work on a project-by-project basis (e.g., Friedland and Kappel, 1979) and that significant sums of money be made available to form interdisciplinary teams to assess the broader social, economic, political, nutritional, food safety, environmental, legal, ethical, and technical issues surrounding the new biotechnologies.

• Partly because of the search for greater value added, and consumer fascination with the new, we are adding complexity to the food production and processing system. In so doing we are exposing the population to new and unknown risks. A more reasonable approach proposed by Knorr and Clancy (1984) is one that asserts the need for minimal rather than maximal processing. That same argument could easily be extended to the entire food and agricultural system. By creating ever more complex dependencies among agriculture and industry, we undermine rather than reinforce our long-term food security both in the United States and throughout the world.

• We also have a responsibility to those who will succeed us in the future. Indeed, this is perhaps the most important issue of all. We all share a desire to leave our progeny a world that is better than the one in which we currently live. This is a noble goal, but it can only be fulfilled by treading lightly and by attempting to see how small increments fit into the larger picture. Our food system is too important to all of us and our progeny to make major changes in it without the broad, democratic participation of all.

It also appears to be appropriate to remember that the annual worldwide budget for biotechnological research does not equal what the nations of the world spend in a week on what is euphemistically called national security. Sad to say, the current definition of national security does not include people's right to food (cf. Busch and Lacy, 1984). If it did, the future would look much brighter indeed.

ACKNOWLEDGMENT

The material in this paper is based on work supported by the National Science Foundation and the National Endowment for the Humanities under grant No. RII-8217306 and the Kentucky Agricultural Experiment Station. We thank Glenn Collins, James Christenson, William H. Friedland, Joan Gussow, David Hildebrande, Richard Merritt, and Louis Swanson for their comments on a previous draft of this paper. Any opinions, findings, conclusions, or recommendations expressed in this publication are those of the authors and do not necessarily reflect the views of the National Science Foundation, the National Endowment for the Humanities, the Kentucky Agricultural Experiment Station, or the reviewers.

REFERENCES

Anderson, L.A., J.D. Phillipson, and M.F. Roberts. 1985. Biosynthesis of secondary products by cell cultures of higher plants. Pp. 1-36 in Plant Cell Culture. Advances in Biochemical Engineering/Biotechnology Series, Vol. 31. Springer-Verlag, New York.

Anonymous. 1986. Cotton fibers grown directly from cells. BOSTID Developments 6(1):12. Board on Science and Technology for International Development, National Research Council, Washington, D.C.

Balandrin, M.F., J.A. Klocke, E.S. Wurtele, and W.H. Bollinger. 1985. Natural plant chemicals: Sources of industrial and medicinal materials. Science 228:1154-1160.

Baltimore, D. 1982. Priorities in biotechnology. Pp. 30-37 in Priorities in Biotechnology Research for International Development: Proceedings of a Workshop. Sponsored by the Board on Science and Technology for International Development held in Washington, D.C. and Berkeley Springs, West Virginia, July 26-30, 1982. National Academy Press, Washington, D.C.

Bijman, J., K. van den Doel, and G. Junne. 1986. The Impact of Biotechnology on Living and Working Conditions in Western Europe and the Third World. European Foundation for the Improvement of Living and Working Conditions, Dublin. 67 pp.

Boyer, C.D. 1984. Genetic engineering: Tomorrow's technology. Am. Veg. Grower 32:51.

Breuling, M., A.W. Alfermann, and E. Reinhard. 1985. Cultivation of cell cultures of Berberis wilsonae in 20-1 airlift bioreactors. Plant Cell Rep. 4:220-223.

Busch, L. 1984. Science, technology, agriculture, and everyday life. Res. Rural Sociol. Dev. 1:289-314.

Busch, L., and W.B. Lacy, eds. 1984. Food Security in the United States. Westview, Boulder, Colo. 452 pp.

Buttel, F.H., and R. Barker. 1985. Emerging agricultural technologies, public policy, and implications for Third World agriculture: The case of biotechnology. Am. J. Agric. Econ. 67:1170-1175.

Byé, P., and A. Mounier. 1984. Les futurs alimentaires et energetiques des biotechnologies. Economies et Sociétés. Hors Serie No. 27. 363 pp.

Chaleff, R.S. 1983. Isolation of agronomically useful mutants from plant cell cultures. Science 219:676-682.

Chamala, S. 1985. Transfer of rubber technology among smallholders in Malaysia and Indonesia: A sociological analysis. Pp. 20-34 in Smallholder Rubber Production and Policies. Australian Centre for International Agricultural Research, Canberra, Australia.

Chatelin, Y. 1986. La science et le developpement: L'histoire peut-elle recommencer? Rev. Tiers Monde 27:5-24.

Chatelin, Y., and R. Arvanitis, eds. 1984. Pratiques et Politiques Scientifiques. Actes du Forum des 6 et 7 Février. Institut Français de Recherche Scientifique pour le Developpement en Cooperation (ORSTOM), Paris.

Clairmonte, F.F., and J. Cavanagh. 1986. Destruction of the sugar industry. Econ. Polit. Weekly 21:18-19.

Collin, H.A., and M. Watts. 1983. Flavor production in culture. Pp. 729-747 in D.A. Evans, W.R. Sharp, P.V. Ammirato, and Y. Yamada, eds. Handbook of Plant Cell Culture, Vol. 1: Techniques for Propagation and Breeding. Macmillan, New York.

Comis, D., and M. Wood. 1986. Assembly line plants take root. Agric. Res. 34:6-11.

Curtin, M.E. 1983. Harvesting profitable products from plant tissue culture. Bio/Technol. 1:649-652, 654, 656-657.

Daly, P. 1985. The Biotechnology Business: A Strategic Analysis. Rowman & Allanheld, Totowa, N.J. 155 pp.

Dembo, D., C. Dias, and W. Morehouse. 1985. The biorevolution and the Third World. Third World Affairs 1:311-325.

Dixon, B. 1984. Chemicals from algae and plant tissue. Bio/Technol. 2:665.

European Economic Community. 1986. Synopsis of Hearing of Biotechnology, 14 January 1986. Directorate General for Research, European Economic Community, Brussels. 15 pp.

FAO (Food and Agriculture Organization). 1985. FAO Trade Yearbook, 1984. Food and Agriculture Organization, Rome. 374 pp.

Fisher, A. 1986. Science Newsfront: Rubber plant. Pop. Sci. 228(5):10.

Fowler, M.W. 1984. Large-scale cultures of cells in suspension. Pp. 167-174 in I.K. Vasil, ed. Cell Culture and Somatic Cell Genetics of Plants. Academic Press, Orlando, Fla.

Friedland, W.H., and T. Kappel. 1979. Production or perish: Changing the inequities of agricultural research priorities. University of California Project on Social Impact Assessment and Values, Santa Cruz, Calif. 40 pp.

Gautheret, R.J. 1983. Plant tissue culture: A history. Bot. Mag. 96:393-410.

Goldstein, D.J. 1988. Molecular biology and the protection of germplasm: A matter of national security. Pp. 315-337 in J. Kloppenburg, Jr., ed. Seeds and Sovereignty: The Use and Control of Plant Genetic Resources. Proceedings of the Annual Meeting of the American Association for the Advancement of Science held in Philadelphia, Pennsylvania, May 25-30, 1986. Duke University Press, Durham, N.C.

Goldstein, W.E. 1983. Large-scale processing of plant cell culture. Ann. N.Y. Acad. Sci. 413:394-408.

Goonatilake, S. 1982. Crippled Minds: An Exploration into Colonial Culture! Vikas, New Delhi, India. 350 pp.

Hansen, M., L. Busch, J. Burkhardt, W.B. Lacy, and L.R. Lacy. 1986. Plant breeding and biotechnology. BioScience 36:29-39.

Heinstein, P.F. 1985. Future approaches to the formation of secondary natural products in plant cell suspension cultures. J. Nat. Prod. 48:1-9.

Ihde, D. 1979. Technics and Praxis. D. Reidel, Dordrecht, Holland. Distributed by Kluwer Academic, Norwell, Mass. 151 pp.

James, A.T. 1984. Plant tissue culture: Achievements and prospects. Proc. R. Soc. London, Ser. B 222:135-145.

Kenney, M., F.H. Buttel, and J. Kloppenburg, Jr. 1984. Impact of industrial applications: Socioeconomic impact of product dislocations. Adv. Technol. Alert Syst. Bull. 1:48-51.

Knorr, D., and K.L. Clancy. 1984. Safety aspects of processed foods. Pp. 231-253 in L. Busch and W.B. Lacy, eds. Food Security in the United States. Westview, Boulder, Colo.

Laudan, R., ed. 1984. The Nature of Technological Knowledge: Are Models of Scientific Change Relevant? D. Reidel, Dordrecht, Holland. Distributed by Kluwer Academic, Norwell, Mass. 145 pp.

Lenin, V.I. 1938. Theory of the Agrarian Question. International Publishers, New York. 335 pp.

Martin-Leake, H. 1975. An historical memoir of the indigo industry in Bihar. Econ. Bot. 29:361-371.

Misawa, M. 1985. Production of useful plant metabolites. Pp. 59-88 in Plant Cell Culture. Advances in Biochemical Engineering/Biotechnology Series, Vol. 31. Springer-Verlag, New York.

Moshy, R. 1986. Biotechnology: Its potential impact on traditional food processing. Pp. 1-14 in S.K. Harlander and T.P. Labuza, eds. Biotechnology in Food Processing. Noyes, Park Ridge, N.J.

Radin, D.N., H.M. Behl, P. Proksch, and E. Rodriquez. 1982. Rubber and other hydrocarbons produced in tissue cultures of guayule (Parthenium argentatum). Plant Sci. Lett. 26:301-310.

Randolph, S.R., and C. Sachs. 1981. The establishment of applied sciences: Medicine and agriculture compared. Pp. 83-111 in L. Busch, ed. Science and Agricultural Development. Allanheld, Osmun, Totowa, N.J.

Rogoff, M.H., and S.L. Rawlins. 1987. Food security: A technological alternative. BioScience 37:800-807.

Ronk, R. 1986. Federal regulation of food biotechnology. Pp. 29-35 in S.K. Harlander and T.P. Labuza, eds. Biotechnology in Food Processing. Noyes, Park Ridge, N.J.

Rosevear, A., and C.A. Lambe. 1985. Immobilized plant cells. Pp. 37-58 in Plant Cell Culture. Advances in Biochemical Engineering/Biotechnology Series, Vol. 31. Springer-Verlag, New York.

Schaeffer, G.W., and F.T. Sharpe, Jr. 1983. Mutations and cell selections: Genetic variations for improved protein in rice. Pp. 237-254 in L.D. Owens, ed. Genetic Engineering: Applications to Agriculture. Symposium held at the Beltsville Agricultural Research Center, Beltsville, Maryland, May 16-19, 1982. Sponsored by the Agricultural Research Service, U.S. Department of Agriculture. Rowman & Allanheld, Totowa, N.J.

Senior, P. 1986. Scale-up of a fermentation process. Pp. 249-257 in S.K. Harlander and T.P. Labuza, eds. Biotechnology in Food Processing. Noyes, Park Ridge, N.J.

Simon, R. 1986. Mail-order enzymes. Forbes 137:46.

Staba, E.J. 1985. Milestones in plant tissue culture systems for the production of secondary products. J. Nat. Prod. 48:203-209.

Stanley, D.W. 1986. Chemical and structural determinants of texture of fabricated foods. Food Technol. 40(3): 65-68, 76.

Tsai, C.H., and J.E. Kinsella. 1981. Initiation and growth of callus and cell suspensions of Theobroma cacao L. Ann. Bot. 48:549-557.

van den Doel, K., and G. Junne. 1986. Product substitution through biotechnology: Impact on the Third World. Trends Biotechnol. 4:88-90.

Vergopoulos, K. 1985. The end of agribusiness or the emergence of biotechnology. Int. Soc. Sci. J. 37:285-299.

Wheat, D. 1986. Strategies for commercialization of biotechnology in the food industry. Pp. 279-284 in S.K. Harlander and T.P. Labuza, eds. Biotechnology in Food Processing. Noyes, Park Ridge, N.J.

Wittwer, S.H. 1985. New technology needed to sustain increased food production. Pp. 1-55 in Food For the Future: The Philadelphia Society for Promoting Agriculture, Bicentennial Forum Proceedings 1785-1985. Philadelphia Society for Promoting Agriculture, Philadelphia.

Yamada, Y. 1984. Selection of cell lines for high yields of secondary metabolites. Pp. 629-636 in I.K. Vasil, ed. Cell Culture and Somatic Cell Genetics of Plants. Academic Press, Orlando, Fla.

Yamada, Y., and Y. Fujita. 1983. Production of useful compounds in culture. Pp. 717-728 in D.A. Evans, W.R. Sharp, P.V. Ammirato, and Y. Yamada, eds. Handbook of Plant Cell Culture, Vol. 1: Techniques for Propagation and Breeding. Macmillan, New York.

Zenk, M. 1978. The impact of plant cell culture on industry. Pp. 1-13 in T.A. Thorpe, ed. Frontiers of Plant Tissue Culture. International Association for Plant Tissue Culture, Calgary, Alberta, Canada.

AUTHORS AND COAUTHORS

LAWRENCE BUSCH, Professor, Department of Sociology, University of Kentucky, Lexington, Kentucky

JACK DOYLE, Director, Agricultural Resources Project, Environmental Policy Institute, Washington, D.C.

ALBERT GORE, JR., U.S. Senator, D-Tennessee

ERNEST G. JAWORSKI, Director, Biological Sciences, Monsanto Company, St. Louis, Missouri

WILLIAM B. LACY, Department of Sociology, Kentucky Agricultural Experiment Station, University of Kentucky, Lexington, Kentucky

ROBERT H. LAWRENCE, JR., Vice President, U.S. Tobacco, Greenwich, Connecticut